Praise for *Parent Goals*

"Garrett rejects the standard of mothers as 'default parents' and writes to parents as a team, offering no shortage of practical advice. New parents will find this [book] worth returning to."

—PUBLISHERS WEEKLY

"If you're considering parenthood, but you're not sure what questions you should be asking, how you should emotionally prepare, or what to do to set yourself up for success, this is the book for you. Garrett's advice is smart, thoughtful, and incredibly useful."

—MELINDA WENNER MOYER, contributing editor, *Scientific American*, and author of *How to Raise Kids Who Aren't Assholes*

"One of the most challenging parts of parenting is dealing with the unknown. *Parent Goals* helps demystify those early days and offers parents concrete advice as they prepare for their new roles. By sharing her own experiences and expertise, Garrett helps parents be thoughtful and purposeful in their parenting decisions."

—DR. CHRISTIA SPEARS BROWN, author of *Parenting Beyond Pink & Blue* and *Unraveling Bias*

"If you're looking for your baby's user manual . . . well, that doesn't exist but *Parent Goals* comes pretty close. Garrett mixes her own story as a mom with her journey as a parenting mental health specialist, and then adds in nuggets of goodness from all the parents she interviewed. *Parent Goals* is a real honest look at preparing for a baby mixed with optimism and humor."

—ROBYN GOBBEL, therapist and parent educator

Parent Goals

Parent Goals

The Millennial's Guide to New Parent Preparedness

Lindsay C.M. Garrett, LCSW

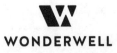

WONDERWELL

Library of Congress Control Number: 2021912216

ISBN 978-1-63756-008-2 (paperback)
ISBN 978-1-63756-009-9 (EPUB)

Editor: Allison Serrell
Cover design and interior design: Morgan Krehbiel
Original cover image: iStock.com/samxmeg
Author photo: EightyTwo Photo

Published by Wonderwell in Los Angeles, CA
www.wonderwell.press

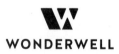

WONDERWELL

Distributed in the US by Publishers Group West and in
Canada by Publishers Group Canada

Printed and bound in Canada

*To John, who partners me in all things,
and to G and R, whose impending
existence caused this book to be written*

Contents

Foreword

AS A PSYCHOLOGIST trained in child development, I felt pretty confident about becoming a parent. I casually read a book about breastfeeding but otherwise approached the birth of my first son with a surprising degree of nonchalance. And then . . . wham! Parenthood hit me square in the face. Everything from a chaotic delivery to feeding challenges to disagreements with my spouse about how to parent made raising this little human feel overwhelming.

None of it was going according to plan! To top it off, the swells of self-doubt that accompanied the chaos prompted a massive identity crisis as my confidence wavered about whether or not I could actually do this. News flash—turns out my biggest challenge was that *I hadn't actually made a plan!* Looking back, I realize I should have spent a lot more time contemplating my parent goals.

But everything happens for a reason, and I now see that this crisis happened *for* me, not *to* me. I had so much to learn about getting my parenting swagger on! Since those early days of motherhood, I've been able to pass along the lessons I learned to the thousands of new parents I've had the privilege to support throughout my twenty-plus-year career. That said, if I could have changed one thing about being a new parent, I would have started the journey a little more eyes-wide-open to minimize the intensity of that precious beginning.

Lindsay C.M. Garrett, LCSW, offers new parents just the kind of clarity and guidance I wish I'd had in this accessible and engaging book. As a mother herself who has spent her career supporting parents through adoption preparation, Lindsay really gets what goes into thinking through the enormous concept of what it is to welcome a child into your life. With personal anecdotes and a healthy dose of humor, Lindsay capably guides hopeful new parents through this monumental life decision, offering a wealth of knowledge, concrete examples, and insightful tips.

One of the things that makes early parenting so challenging is that there is a sort of mythical assumption about how warm and fuzzy it all ought to feel. The reality is often very different. And yet, because of stigma, we often don't talk about the hard parts, opting instead to just keep our heads down and tough it out. Lindsay is real about the mess and the challenges, and her voice throughout *Parent Goals* offers steady assurance that this is all normal.

In my work as a psychologist, I often find myself wishing I had a how-to guide to give to clients who are contemplating parenthood or who find themselves feeling a little lost in those early days and months of being a parent. *Parent Goals* is that guide. As someone who reads most of the new parenting books published each year, I can confidently tell you this is the one I have been waiting for.

Dr. Vanessa Lapointe, registered psychologist and author of the bestselling *Discipline Without Damage* and award-winning *Parenting Right From the Start*.

Introduction

I N THE SUMMER of 2016, my husband, John, and I were eleven years into our friendship, four years into our romantic relationship, and had been married just shy of one year. Natives of Fort Worth, Texas, we had recently relocated to Houston—a terrifying and unknown leap into a new adventure—and had just begun to discuss another terrifying and unknown leap: having children (*dun dun dun!*).

John and I met as summer camp counselors and had seen each other in action with children, so this area was not a great mystery for either of us. We'd had the "hypothetical kid" discussion even before we got married. We both wanted kids: two, maybe three. John had made several jokes throughout the conversation about how the men in his family father only boys, so we wouldn't possibly have any girls (cue eye roll from me) . . . and so on.

Being type A and Enneagram Type 1 (a.k.a. a perfectionist) *and* a mental health professional, I have an innate desire to overmanage pretty much everything. Before taking a leap, I must do the research and talk about all the possible outcomes. Pro and con lists are required. Information is to me like drugs to an addict; I cannot get enough. Spreadsheets are a facet of my daily stress management. I know: I am super fun to be married to! To give you some context, when John and I got married, I took the lead on planning our wedding and . . . *enjoyed it*. A year before that I was by my best friend/sister-in-law's side as she planned her own wedding and was offered two wedding planner jobs in the process. This is my gift. Or my downfall, depending on how you see it.

When John and I were dating and began discussing engagement, I came home with a book titled something like *One Hundred and One Questions to Ask before Marriage*, and we read through it together. While we were engaged, we went to a church-mandated marriage preparation course (extraneous for us; but alas, Catholic hoops) and also attended marriage preparation sessions with a counselor. I read books about the sociological ramifications of marriage; I followed blogs about marriage, weddings, and relationships in general. We were *prepared*. The day we said "I do," I had no qualms at all. At the very least, I reasoned, the man who had calmly and optimistically indulged me in all of these preparations was certainly well suited to partner me through all the other unknowns life brings, and would remain by my side as I systematically researched and made lists about each and every one of them.

While on our honeymoon in September 2015, John got an email that would turn our lives upside down. He had been accepted into a training program to become an air traffic controller (if you don't know what that is, watch the movie *Pushing Tin*). Four months later he moved to Oklahoma City to begin training while I stayed in Fort Worth, and four months after that, we were packing to move to Houston for John's new job. While the move was not as far as it could have been, it was the first time both of us would relocate hours away from all of our family and friends. For me, at least, that was a big deal.

Throughout all of this change, we continued our discussions about having children. By the time we moved I was on the verge of thirty and felt a sense of urgency that I think may be familiar for many women this age who have not yet had children but also haven't ruled out doing so. For me, this urgency took the form of a not-so-subtle alarm in my head that said, *Let's get this show on the road! You only have a few years left before all of your eggs jump ship! Hurry, Hurry, Hurry!* At the same time, I did not feel a huge yearning for a baby. I pictured our future with children, and I knew that I planned to have them, but I didn't have the "baby fever" I saw in some of my friends.

Naturally, when John and I started to discuss the timing of having children, I did what I always do. I took to the internet to gather any knowledge that I could. I found books and articles about what to expect during pregnancy, planning financially for a child, fertility, questions to ask your doctor, and how to care for babies. But in this deluge of data, I didn't find exactly what I was looking for. I wanted something similar to the marriage preparation we undertook to help us plan for the transition, discuss challenges, and explore issues we were likely to encounter before we got there. I wanted a list of questions we should ask each other before becoming parents, suggestions on ways to prepare for our new roles and responsibilities, and a heads-up on conflicts that might arise. But it just didn't exist. When I lamented this void to my best friend, she said, "I bet you could write something like that." I laughed it off at the time, but then found I couldn't shake the idea. As I continued to contemplate all of the issues I wanted to explore before embarking on parenthood, I realized she might be right.

After all, I am a licensed clinical social worker, and I have a master of science in social work with a focus on children and families. I've worked in the adoption field for nearly ten years, and my entire job focuses on parenting readiness. I've worked with families adopting newborns, adopting from other countries, and adopting from foster care, and I've counseled couples who have experienced infertility. In addition to conducting home study assessments to ensure families are prepared for parenting, I help support them through the waiting process before they become parents. I facilitate trainings on parent preparedness that cover topics including attachment styles, discipline strategies, infant brain development, and self-care. I also support families post-adoption in dealing with concerning behaviors in their child or conflicts in their marriage that arise as a result of parenting, and help them find resources in their community. I have extensive training in trauma, child development, attachment, grief and loss, and identity, and I teach parents how to have difficult conversations with their child about these issues. I've seen what works to make parents successful, and what contributes to additional struggles or failures. Between my job and my role as the mother of two small children, I am, on a daily basis, knee-deep in the nitty-gritty of parenting and how to prepare for it.

During the pre-adoption trainings I give, I often hear comments from parents like, "I wish I had known this before my biological children were born" or "We wish we had talked about this before we had kids." (Since our training is primarily geared toward families adopting older children, attendees were often already parents before they decided to adopt.) Here are a few of the topics parents said they wished they had known about before they had kids:

- The importance of self-care for parents, and how caring for yourself directly benefits your children.

- That you don't have to be a perfect parent. Getting things wrong and making mistakes is often an opportunity to make a repair that leads to greater connection with your child.
- That it's important to look at your history with your own parents and how that can affect your parenting and your interactions with your children. We parent the way we were parented unless we take active and intentional steps to change that.
- How the infant brain develops, and how to maximize the impact of child interactions to gain connection and compliance.

Overall, the parents I see wish they'd had some sense of what they were getting themselves into beyond the glib "Oh, you'll see" or "Wait until *you* become a parent" comments so often delivered by seasoned parents to non-parents. Hearing this from clients over and over, I knew that others would benefit from this knowledge as well. After some brainstorming and a successful talk with John, where he once again agreed to indulge me on my journey, the idea of writing this book began to take shape.

A little bit more about me: I am squarely in the range of "elder millennial," which means I didn't have the internet for my entire life and I still remember things like cassette tapes, VHS, and TV shows you could not rewind. I toe the line between embracing technology and resisting it (I am still trying to keep up with Instagram but I think Snapchat is a scam). I love me some avocado toast, but I think participation trophies are stupid. And, like many millennials, I took the decision to have a kid very, very seriously.

We millennials are the generation born between 1981 and 1996. As of this writing in 2020, we are between the ages of twenty-four and thirty-nine and are currently the largest generation in history, surpassing even baby boomers (okay, boomer). Research indicates that my generation is pretty cautious about becoming parents.[1] In 2016, the average mother's age at a first-time birth was 26.4 years, compared with 22.7 in 1980.[2] A 2018 report from the Centers for Disease Control and Prevention showed that birth rates decreased by 2 percent from 2017, noting that 2018 marked the fourth year in a row that birth rates declined. Not only that, but the numbers reached a low not seen since 1986, which is, coincidentally, also the year I was born.[3] Finally, while we millennials are delaying parenting, we are also taking it more seriously than ever before. A Pew Research survey in 2010 found that 57 percent of millennials rated being a good parent as a top priority in their lives, **ahead of having a successful marriage**. In a 2015 survey, also by Pew, 60 percent identified being a parent as extremely important to their overall identity.[4]

Where our parents may have considered this life stage as "having kids," we are "becoming parents." We see parenting as a verb, a job to do well, a thing to get right—not just something we do because everyone else is doing it, or because it's the presumed "next step" in life. For millennials, it is not just a matter of bringing home a baby, feeding them, sending them outside to play, and trusting that everything will turn out okay. We want to raise children who are emotionally literate, educated on issues of social justice, politically involved, well-read, and can code in their sleep. We are raising a generation that can change the world. I think we can all agree that the pressure is *on*. So, I figured that if I wanted some sort of guide to help me prepare for parenthood, one that included the discussions to have, plans and decisions to make, and potential challenges to explore, perhaps other millennials would be interested as well.

This book is intended to be the guide I didn't have. The information here is taken from my decade of professional experience, all the books and articles I have devoured in my quest to become a well-informed and prepared parent (you're welcome!), and my own experience as the mother of a three-year-old and an eight-month-old.

Though I started off with the idea of sharing my own experiences, I quickly realized that I wanted to include the perspectives of other parents as well. Parenting can be lonely, especially in this day and age when most of us have moved away from our families and live out a significant portion of our lives on social media. I wanted you to hear from other parents—real parents, not influencers on Instagram who are curating their lives to sell you things—that you are not alone. We all get peed on at least once. We all lose sleep. We all wonder, most of the time, what the fuck we are even doing. I included a variety of experiences from different parents with the hope that you will connect with at least one of them.

I interviewed fifty parents, most by phone, and some through a written questionnaire. I specifically targeted parents who identified as millennials or fell within that generation's age range. I also sought out dads, since most of the material in the parenting world is written from the perspective of moms. I interviewed thirty-four moms and sixteen dads. Forty-eight of my interviewees were married and two were single. Their ages ranged from twenty-eight to thirty-eight; the majority were between thirty and thirty-five. Thirty-six of my interviewees were White, eight were African American/Black, one was African, two were Vietnamese, one was Mexican American, one was Latinx, and one was White/Asian. Twenty had more than one child, and thirty had only one child. Their children ranged in age from five months to thirteen years; the majority had children under six. All except one identified as heterosexual, and all identified as cisgender. Six experienced some form of infertility or difficulty conceiving and two had experienced the loss of a child. Forty-one had planned pregnancies, nine had at least one unplanned pregnancy, and three were foster or adoptive parents.

While I hit some of my target interview goals, there are obviously gaps in my data collection. The majority of the parents I interviewed were White and most of them were married. Only one was LGBTQ+, although the spouse of one interviewee was a trans man. Despite my best efforts, the number of moms I interviewed was double the number of dads. I found that few dads were willing to be interviewed on their own (compared to moms, who seemed more than happy to talk about their experience), and that several of them participated at their partner's insistence. I have a few theories about the reasons behind this. As a society, we don't ask for dad's stories as often or make space for them in the parenting world, so they may be less willing to share. Also, in many of the families I spoke with, mom was the default or primary parent, so her experience was much more involved than dad's. There were one or two dads who said that their lives didn't really change that much since becoming a parent (which seemed *unfathomable* to me). Not one of the moms I spoke with said anything remotely similar. This was not a formal study; I simply talked with other parents and collected their stories. I hope you might relate to some of them.

I realize that as a White middle-class mom, my perspective and experience is limited, and hopefully hearing from others will help broaden that a bit. The parents I spoke with were open and vulnerable and many seemed eager to share their experiences with those coming down the path behind them. Parents are the busiest category of people I know, but they carved out time for me in between work, daycare pickup, and caring for their children. I did interviews during naps, in the evenings after kiddos were in bed, and with the constant interruptions that small children bring to any conversation. One particularly delightful moment came when a mom's elegantly insightful statement about the advice she would give herself if she could go back to before she was a parent was capped by her three-year-old proudly announcing, "Mommy I pooped!" If *that* doesn't define parenthood, I don't know what does.

This book is for anyone who is thinking of starting the journey to parenthood or has already started and wants to dig deeper into the preparation process. It is for moms, dads, LGBTQ+ people, nonbinary people, and anyone else who wants to explore this topic. I've tried to keep the language as neutral as possible so that a variety of readers can relate to it. I especially wanted to include information that is relevant to both moms and dads, since so much of the existing parenting literature seems to focus on moms. While this book is written with couples in mind, it can also be explored on your own if you are a single parent or planning to become one. Many of the questions and topics are best to discuss before your child arrives, but several will be useful and relevant for your entire life as a parent.

How to Use This Book

You can read this book from beginning to end, or flip to the most pressing topic for you and start there. Ideally, you and your partner will both read a chapter to get a sense of the topic and then follow the discussion prompts at the end. The end of each chapter includes a summary for those of you who may be more skimmers than readers, or to refresh your memory before diving into the discussion questions. You might read a chapter a week and schedule a time to have an uninterrupted conversation about the topic that is covered. You might each write thoughts down as you go and share them with each other. You could even buy a journal for this exploration, and write down thoughts to each other, passing the journal back and forth if you find writing more comfortable than talking face-to-face. This is a nice way to document the process together, as it is the last time you will be just a duo (as I'm sure you can imagine, things get way more hectic once you have kids). Since I will also give you prompts throughout the book for making specific plans, having a place where you can write them down to refer to later—when you are in the trenches—can help keep you on track. In addition, you'll also find checklists to help you flesh out future plans, and journal prompts for going deeper on topics that may call for more internal exploration.

However you choose to experience this book, at the end of it you will have had some important conversations you likely would not have had otherwise, made practical plans for things like finances and self-care, and set expectations for parenting roles and discipline strategies. My hope is that you will feel just slightly more prepared for the huge life change of becoming parents. Although we all know that there is no way to be fully prepared for jumping into the deep end of parenting, that doesn't mean we shouldn't do everything we can to make ourselves ready. The beauty and challenge of children is that they are constantly changing and growing, and we as parents must evolve right along with them. Ready to get started? Deep breath. Here we go.

So You Think You Want to Be a Parent?

"Parenting was much easier when
I was raising my non-existent
kids hypothetically."

—UNKNOWN

I FEEL LIKE IN every TV comedy featuring a pre-adoption home study there is a social worker who comes into a family's home with white gloves to test for cleanliness, and inevitably something really wacky goes wrong. Okay, I am mainly thinking about the episode of *Friends* where Monica and Chandler are looking to adopt, and it turns out their home study social worker slept with Joey. Don't even get me started on the ethics of *that*.

But seriously, I am truly in awe of the process adoptive parents go through. First, they do a boatload of paperwork, including submitting to background checks, writing mini autobiographies that give their entire life story in a few pages, and filling out medical history forms listing the medications they take and past surgeries or illnesses (in addition to undergoing medical exams). They have to fill out forms about the background of the child they are open to adopting, choosing race, medical history, and mental health history. They have to submit a detailed floor plan and photos of their home, financial records, divorce records, and counseling records. They have to have been married for at least a year, sometimes longer depending on where they are adopting from. Only then are they deemed cleared for the home study visits.

A home study is a full assessment of a family, the goal of which is to identify their strengths, pinpoint any risks they may have, and determine if they are prepared to parent the child they intend to adopt. Compare that to what most families who have a child through pregnancy go through, which is . . . *nothing*. Imagine if you had to bare your soul to a stranger to get permission to have a child, and that the stranger held the power to decide whether or not you were ready. Let's role-play for a moment: "Hi, I'm Lindsay, and I'll be doing your home study today. Please tell me about every hard thing that has ever happened in your life from childhood until now and then let's discuss the risks those events may pose to your parenting." I'm embellishing a bit, but that is not far off the mark. I go deep with families about the trauma they may have experienced in their lives surrounding challenges like divorce, addiction, mental health issues, and abusive relationships. And all of that is before we even dive into talking about their marriage.

The really remarkable thing about doing home studies is that I have the privilege of seeing behind the mask that most people show to the world. My job is to make people feel comfortable enough to share their vulnerabilities with me. I factor those into the bigger picture of their future parenting journey and help them identify what might be a struggle down the road; I also help them see what wonderful strengths they will bring to the table as parents. Essentially, we conduct these home studies to determine if a family is ready for the momentous job and commitment of parenting. At the end of the day, we do it all for the child. If I have parents who aren't on the same page about adopting, or who don't understand exactly what the job entails, or who are still trying to work through some marital conflict or past personal trauma, then ultimately, it's going to be the child who suffers. We know from research that what a parent brings to the table emotionally directly affects their child, adopted or not.

If you've picked up this book, you likely care very deeply about the decision to become a parent. It is important to you that you set your family up for success. That's exactly what I do for my adoptive parents, and what I can help you do too. If you're feeling a bit overwhelmed right now, try not to fret. One of the things about parenting is that there is an overwhelming amount of information out there, and it's sometimes difficult to know what is important and what is not. That's where I come in. I'm going to cut through the clutter to teach you what you need to know. We'll look at your own history and how that might affect your expectations and parenting style. Together, we'll create a strategy for how to get ready. In a nutshell, you'll have a plan before your child arrives, and this will be something you can refer to in those early parenting days and reflect on throughout your life as a parent.

As I outlined earlier, families who pursue adoption jump through a lot of hoops. But they do it because they have such a strong desire to become parents. I imagine you might feel the same way. Or maybe you picked this book up because you aren't sure you want to be a parent and want to get a sense of what you might be in for. Both of these reasons are a great place to start.

Begin at the Beginning

The first thing to do when thinking about becoming a parent is to start talking about it with your partner, assuming you are doing this as a couple. I usually ask the families I work with this question: "What makes you want to be a parent in the first place?" It's a solid start to any discussion with your partner on this topic. I'll explore this question in more detail later in the chapter, but before we get there, we need to decide *if* you want to be a parent. And if you have a partner, do they want to be one too? I typically ask couples to each rate their desire to become parents, and we can do the same here: "On a scale of one to ten, how would you rate your personal desire to be a parent?"

You and your partner can answer this separately, perhaps writing your number down and then showing the other. This will help you both do some personal reflection and decide where you feel you are at on this scale without influence from the other. From there you can have a conversation about where each of you landed. When I do this with parents, I usually get at least one person who tells me they are an eleven or twelve, meaning they really, really want to be a parent. But I also get people who say they are an eight or a nine, and occasionally a seven. When that happens, my question to them is "What keeps you from being a ten?" If they aren't feeling a strong desire to become a parent, or excitement at the prospect, what might be holding them back? Often it is a specific fear, or just general anxiety about the unknown. (Don't worry, we have an entire chapter devoted to fears coming up.) But sometimes it might be that they don't actually know if they want to be a parent, or they know they don't want to, but their partner desperately wants a child, and they want to make their partner happy. This is where we get into some tricky territory, and I want to make something very clear before we go any further. I say this to you as you start down this path, kindly but clearly (as shame researcher and my general idol Brené Brown tells us to):

If you are not both on board with becoming parents, it will erode and damage your relationship, your marriage, and eventually your family that you worked so hard to create.

I have seen this happen. Parenting is magical and wondrous, but it is also stressful and a constant challenge. If you are not both up for tackling the challenge together, it is going to be much harder. Depending on where you both are on the scale, you can discuss what might be holding you back. In fact, I suggest you write these thoughts down so you can refer to them throughout the book. There may be many things holding you back from full-on commitment; you might be worried about how your career fits into parenting, or just generally fearful of how the hell you're going to keep a tiny human alive. We're going to cover these fears in chapter 3, but for now, let's forge ahead.

Assuming you want to be a parent at least a little bit, I am now going to revisit my first question: "What makes you want to be a parent in the first place?" The answer is probably a little different for everyone. Some people have a passion for children and want to share their love with a child. Some want to pass on their family traditions or name, and some want to experience the joys of parenthood with their spouse. Alternatively, one partner could be on board because the other desperately wants to be a mom or a dad, and while they are on the fence, they want to make their partner happy, so they go along with it. Sometimes potential parents think a child will be a fresh start, perhaps a haven from the tumultuous or traumatic childhood they experienced. It can be one reason, or many all tied up together. This is another good question to reflect on, write about in your journal, and refer to later on.

Looking through Your Partner's Eyes

When deciding to take on the adventure of parenthood together, knowing your partner's motivation can help you to see things from their point of view and make you more compassionate if they are struggling with a particular aspect of becoming a parent. This can deepen your relationship and also help you both set expectations about specific aspects of raising children. Expectations are *huge* influencers on how the transition to becoming parents will go, and if they are unrealistic, it can increase the likelihood that you may struggle more or can potentially contribute to mental health conditions. Maybe your partner wants to be a parent in order to pass on their family legacy, or to see you become a parent as well. Maybe they want to be a parent because they think they are supposed to, or because of pressure from their own parents. All of these potential reasons are important to articulate up front.

When I considered my own reasons for wanting to be a parent, my first thought was how I find such joy in my interactions with children. Although I was an only child, I babysat from my preteen years on, I was a camp counselor, and I had dozens of cousins to play with growing up. I feel like I just light up around children. They are fascinating and funny and unapologetically themselves. I love children so much that I decided to spend my career striving to improve their lives. While I think children are a joy to be with and play with, I didn't feel a strong pull toward having a child until I was almost thirty and had been married for a year or so. At that point, small pangs of longing would sneak up on me when meeting a friend's new baby or playing a game with my godson. I would feel a rush of love and think, *I could do this.*

When I asked John why he wanted to be a parent, his answer surprised me. I expected to hear something about continuing the family bloodline or just creating that family he pictured having somewhere down the road. He said his motivation was the experience of parenthood itself. He felt that being a parent helps you to grow as an individual, and he wanted to see our future children grow as well. He also noted our close relationships with our parents as something he hoped to experience with our own children one day. We are both fortunate to have close-knit families and enjoy spending time with our parents and other relatives.

On Different Pages

What if you and your partner's motivations don't line up? Let's look at an example:

Ashley was on the fence about having children when she and her husband got married. They had agreed to wait until they had been married for five years to have kids, and she genuinely believed she would feel differently when they reached that milestone. She felt she married young and thought as she got older the desire to be a parent would grow. Cut to their five-year anniversary. Ashley found herself putting up all sorts of barriers for her and her husband when it came to being "ready" to be parents. These included things like losing weight, putting finances in order, planning all the trips they wouldn't be able to take once they had children, and making sure everything was "just right." After many arguments and more than a few counseling sessions, she and her husband dove deeper into how they were each feeling. It came down to this: he wanted to have a biological child and wanted his wife to be pregnant and birth that child. The biological tie was very important to him, as was having a baby. Ashley had no desire at all to be pregnant or give birth, and the biological component was not important to her. She was not particularly interested in babies and would rather have adopted an elementary school–aged child. They ended up compromising and adopting a two-year-old. Neither seemed particularly happy about the compromise.

Should they have had this conversation earlier? Maybe. How will this affect their child? That remains to be seen. Regardless, entering parenthood is by itself a gamble, and going in when you're not in agreement with your partner decreases the odds of success. According to the Gottman Institute, an organization that helps struggling couples reconnect through research, tools, and interventions, two out of three marriages decrease in satisfaction after the addition of a child.[5] Combine that with potential conflict or resentment toward your partner and you have a recipe for an ongoing struggle at best.

Let's look at one other couple. Mia got married in her early thirties and was undecided about having children. She and her fiancée discussed it before getting married and it was clear that her fiancée really wanted kids. Mia was a devoted partner who desired to make her fiancée happy, so she agreed to have at least one child after they were married. She thought her love for her partner and desire to see her happy would be motivation enough. A couple of years into their marriage, they decided to begin their journey of trying to get pregnant. Just a few weeks in, Mia found herself panicking. She was deeply unhappy and could not pinpoint the source. She distanced herself from her wife, friends, and family. She and her wife started going to therapy. Mia discovered that when push came to shove, she could not go through with having a child just to make her wife happy. What started with the best of intentions and love for her spouse resulted in the end of their marriage.

The upshot here is that parenting is hard and is not to be taken lightly. It is an all-encompassing job that affects every member of your family. I've seen families who had cracks in their marriage that could be ignored until the added stress of parenting brought them to the surface, and then they had to try to repair their marriage while also figuring out how to be parents together. I've seen parents who have unresolved trauma or emotional baggage that is triggered by their child. Some can work through it. But some can't, and that leads to their family falling apart or them blaming their child for everything they are feeling. Imagine being that child.

Another thing to note is that if you go the pregnancy route to becoming parents, the reality is that in the beginning a lot of the work falls on the person who is pregnant, and if you add breastfeeding to the mix, that work continues for a year or more. You have to really be on board to go through it. While I like to advocate for equal participation from both parents as much as possible in all aspects of parenting, this area really becomes lopsided for a while for many couples, especially heterosexual ones where the woman carries and births the baby. If the spouse who is biologically predestined to take on those responsibilities is not on board, it is a lot harder to soldier through. I've seen several different-sex families where mom becomes the primary parent and dad participates when he wants—a choice the mother simply does not have in those first years when a baby may be relying on her for comfort and nourishment. This dynamic could obviously be different in relationships where spouses are of the same sex, and there are of course things like formula feeding, childcare, and support that can mitigate the burden.

What Other Parents Said

You may not know the exact reasons you want to be a parent at this point, which is why I asked parents "What made you want to be a parent?" during my interviews. I thought their answers might inspire you. I got a lot of responses that were a version of "I always knew I wanted to be a parent," particularly from the moms I interviewed. My hypothesis on this is that our society tells women they should all be mothers at some point during their lives, but since I don't have valid data to support that, and we could spend an entire book talking about the patriarchy, I won't go down that particular rabbit hole now. Here's what my interviewees said about why they wanted to be parents:

A LOVE OF CHILDREN

"I always wanted to be a parent. Babies and kids were a huge part of my life growing up and I loved being around them."

"I have always been the responsible person who loves taking care of people. I have a brother who is twelve years younger than me, so I helped care for him. I love taking care of kids. Friends would joke about me wanting to steal babies. I find joy in caring for them and watching them grow and I love seeing life through their eyes."

"I like interacting with kids. I thought it would be a fun, different adventure. I wanted to burn some money and lose some sleep."

"I've always been around children. My mom and I took in a lot of kids who were in need. I was sixteen when a set of twins were born, and we took them in. From them on I knew that I wanted to be a mom."

"I always saw myself with kids, although I didn't know what that would look like. I knew I wanted to enjoy the things I liked in my childhood with my kids."

"I always thought I would be a dad at some point. I felt like life would be empty later if you didn't have kids."

KIDS AS A NEXT STEP

"I was twenty-eight and hearing about others who had struggled getting pregnant. We knew we wanted a big family, so we decided to start. We were at a good place financially and felt stable."

"It just felt like that next logical step for me. I didn't necessarily feel ready for it or an urge to be a father, or that my life was missing something. I thought it would be interesting to have a child to pass things down to. It seemed like a natural progression in planning for the future."

"We felt like the world needed our genes. It seemed like the next step and gave us meaning."

"We both knew we needed to get to a certain point before adding a child to that. We probably talked for six months before starting to try. We knew we would be bringing a child into a bigger extended family that was all nearby, so it was easier to make that decision because I knew we had that support system."

"In my head I've always wanted to be a mom, and we decided it was right for us to become parents when we were settled as far as finances go, we were in good places in our careers, etc."

"Coming from a big family it was like autopilot. You get married, you have children."

"After we were married for a few years it felt like we were there in our relationship and marriage and ready to complete our family. I felt ready to be a dad, and I've always wanted to be a father."

"I always wanted to be a parent. Growing up in a Mexican household I have a lot of cousins, and I am the oldest of three. I always knew I wanted to be a mom."

CONTRIBUTING TO THE WORLD

"I also feel like one way we make a better world is through raising children well, and I wanted to do my part in that. It's hard to think societal pressure wasn't also a factor in some sense."

"I have great parents, and I grew up in an environment where critical thought, and also expression of love and affection, were encouraged. I always hoped that I would be able to pass those ideals on to another generation."

"There was a moment in my life where I made the decision that starting a family was one of the most unequivocally good things you could do in this world. One of the many ways we make the world a better place is to raise happy, well-adjusted kids."

GIVING WHAT THEY DIDN'T GET

"I have always wanted to be a better parent than I had. My parents did what they could, but there were struggles."

"I wanted to have a family with my significant other, and I wanted the family I never grew up having as an only child."

"I thought being a dad would be really cool, and I wanted to contribute to a life and give my child a better life than I had."

"It was always just a given for me. I always wanted kids, played house, and wanted to have a family. A big part of it was being able to see if I could do something different than what my parents provided and thinking this could be kind of a cool experiment. I felt like I could do a good job."

UNSURE ABOUT BEING A PARENT

"I wasn't sure that I wanted to be a parent. I took care of my niece when I was in high school, so I knew how to change diapers and things like that. I didn't know that I wanted to be a parent until I had my own kid. The feeling is like no other. It's a part of you—and once they can show that love to you it is another level; it's like a high."

"I wasn't sure I wanted to be a parent when I was in my early twenties. Being with my now-husband and seeing how amazing he is with kids was the only thing that made me want to be a parent at first. I wanted to make him a dad because I knew he'd be amazing at it. After we got married and as others around us started having children, I really wanted it. I wanted to experience pregnancy and help my own child grow and learn. I wanted my husband and I to have a little one to shower our love on and share experiences with."

"I am not the one who grew up thinking, When I grow up, I am going to be a mom. *I also never saw myself being a stay-at-home mom. I knew it was always part of a plan that sounded fine by me, and I've always loved working with kids."*

"Working with animals, I see a lot of really horrible people, and I was really back and forth on whether I wanted to have a child in a world where people are that terrible. My own family and the relationship I have with my parents and brother now made me want to. I wanted to keep my family going and have those times together with our children."

———

Keep in mind that all of the people I interviewed were already parents, and their comments are reflections on the past. Yes, most of them felt a strong desire to be parents, but it's possible some of them are rewriting history now that they have kids. It's hard to admit that you might not have wanted this phenomenal little being that is now in front of you relying on you for their every need and is freaking adorable at least some of the time. We don't really give parents permission to say things like that; the assumption is that it makes them bad parents, ergo, bad people. Have you ever heard a parent complain about their kid and then immediately follow it up with "But I love them so much!"? As if the fact that they are complaining about how hard it is to be a parent cancels out the love they have for their child. Parents tend to do that. Even so, several of my interviewees expressed uncertainty around parenting, and at least one said they weren't sure about it until their child arrived.

What if one of you is on board to be a parent and the other is unsure? My best advice is to explore what is underneath your reasons. If you or your partner is on the fence, what is underneath that ambivalence? Are you worried about having less time for yourself? Did you have a rough childhood and therefore don't think you would be a good parent? Whatever it is, bring it out into the open so you can work through it together. This would be a great topic to explore with a counselor if you are open to it. A professional therapist or counselor is a neutral party who can help you both express what is going on and guide you to a decision. When looking for a mental health professional, you want to make sure they are licensed in your state, that they have experience working with couples at your stage of life and with your background, and that you have a good connection with them. I recommend setting up phone calls to get a feel for that before you meet in person. Finding a counselor who works for you is kind of like dating. You often have to go on a few first dates to see what clicks. If your partner is reluctant about counseling, you can ask them to try it, setting a boundary of one or two sessions as a trial period and then check in from there. It can also be helpful to ask your partner what makes them hesitant about seeing a professional; they may feel there is a stigma involved or worry about being vulnerable with a stranger. Counseling can seem formidable, especially if you have never done it before. But establishing that connection and knowing it is there *before* the baby arrives and you jump on a one-way train to chaosville is typically much more manageable than researching and calling people once you are in the trenches of parenthood.

If you or your partner aren't sure, need more time, or feel like you don't want children, that is completely valid. You just might not want to spend your time reading an entire book about preparing to be a parent if that's the case, which is why we start this conversation here in chapter 1.

Diving into the Deep End

The discussion of whether or not to have children can be a big eye-opener or even throw a wrench in your plans, depending on how you both feel, so I urge you to get clarity on this issue now.

Assuming you will change your opinion down the road, or that your partner will, or that you can suck it up and have kids just for them are all dangerous gambles. It's best to tackle these issues ahead of time, not when you are sleep-deprived at 2 a.m. thinking, *What the hell did I get myself into?* If you and your partner are on the same page about your desires to be parents, congratulations! That is a great first step. There is much more to explore, so buckle up and get ready to roll.

Summary

- Starting your parenting discussion by asking each other why you want to be parents helps identify your motivations and any differing inclinations you may have about having children.

- If you are not both on board with being parents there is a strong likelihood this will erode and damage your relationship, your marriage, and eventually the family you worked to create.

- Knowing your partner's "why" behind becoming a parent can foster compassion, help deepen your relationship, and set expectations for the future.

- If you go the pregnancy route to parenting, know that whoever carries and births the baby is likely going to end up doing more of the work, especially in the first year.

- There are many valid reasons for wanting to be a parent, but it is also normal to be unsure and need more time to decide before making this lifelong commitment.

- If you run into some hard or sticky conversations during this discussion or throughout the course of reading this book, consider seeing a counselor to help you and your partner navigate those challenges.

Discussion Topics:
Motivation

1. What makes each of you want to be a parent?

2. Rate both of your desires to be parents on a scale of one to ten.

3. What is the reason behind your rating? Do either of you rate your desire higher than the other?

4. Are your reasons for wanting to be parents different? Were you surprised by your answers?

5. How do you feel your motivations may come into play when you are in the trenches of parenthood?

6. Do you have any concerns you may need to discuss with a therapist?

7. Do you feel like you are on the same page about your decision to become parents?

It's All in the Timing

"'We must hurry!' said Mr. Wonka. 'We have so much time and so little to do! No! Wait! Strike that! Reverse it!'"

—ROALD DAHL

MY MOM WAS pregnant with me at the age of twenty-one. I didn't think much about that age until I reached it myself and realized how absolutely insane it would be for me to have a kid at that time in my life. I was in college and grad school, working part-time jobs to make ends meet, with growing student loan debt and a ramen-for-dinner budget. When I made it to twenty-two still baby free, I felt I had somehow dodged a bullet.

Timing is everything, right? Now that you've decided you want to start down the path to parenthood, or are at least seriously considering it, it's time to look at the *when* and *how*. In this chapter I'll guide you through three of the most important factors in determining the right time to have kids: feeling ready, finances, and your path to parenthood. This is where we get down to business.

I think we can all agree that timing when to have a child

is a modern-day luxury for those of us with access to decent healthcare. I spent my twenties *very actively* avoiding pregnancy, and after I got married, I was relieved to have made it to some imagined "safe place" where if I did unexpectedly get pregnant there would be less perceived social stigma. I felt as if I'd already roped someone into being in the mess of life with me, so if an unplanned pregnancy happened, we would at least be in it together. That somehow seemed less scary.

John and I had already settled on starting with pregnancy as our preferred method of bringing a child into our family. I had several reservations surrounding pregnancy (see the next chapter on fears) but was willing to try it out. We were in prime childbearing age; we had the biological parts to make and birth a baby; we lived in a city with great medical care; we were both pretty healthy; and we thought a mash-up of our genes might come out cute. This seemed a good fit for us, assuming we were able to conceive. Working at an adoption agency, I frequently interacted with couples who experienced infertility, which means I had a healthy dose of skepticism around pregnancy happening naturally or easily. For John, having a biological child was important, as he felt it would allow him to attach and bond to our child more easily (this was literally the most convincing argument he could have made, since I am obsessed with attachment theory, which we'll discuss in chapter 6). I didn't have strong feelings about adoption versus biological children. We discussed possibly adopting in the future, but for now, we were going to try the old-fashioned way. I felt like pregnancy would never win in a pro-versus-con list of whether to try it, but then again, neither would adoption. Both can be challenging and joyful. It seems that sacrifice is required no matter which way you bring children into your family. I still can't decide if that is poetic or terrible, so let's go with poetic and lean toward the positive, shall we?

We began our more serious discussions about family planning during the summer and had set a tentative time of January to begin trying to get pregnant. Side note: If you are starting these conversations, this is a good time to get agreement about what "trying to get pregnant" means for you. For us, it meant tossing the contraception and seeing what came of it. This lasted all of a hot second before I was obsessively tracking my cycles and pinpointing ovulation dates on the calendar. I stopped short of examining my cervical mucus daily—mostly because it grossed me out. But hey, you do you if that's your thing.

I had mixed feelings about our start date. While I was feeling little pangs of "I could have a baby," by no means did I feel a strong craving or pull toward having one right that minute, or even in the timeline we were talking about. With further personal reflection and discussion with John, I realized I would never feel totally ready to take that leap. As previously stated, I am a planner and I like to have things in order and under my control. Pregnancy and birth took all of that away from me, and there was no getting around it. In the end, it seemed that this timing was as good as any. As for John, he was looking ahead to the future, calculating what age we could be when our children graduated from high school, college, and maybe had children of their own. These are all events we wanted to be around and—the universe willing—in good health for. So that was that. We made the decision to start trying at the beginning of the following year, and even threw out a few jokes about unprotected New Year's Eve sex. Spoiler: This did not happen; I spent New Year's Eve with my head in a trash can. I had decided to have one last night of drinking, since I'd be avoiding alcohol for the next two years. I have no regrets. And no, you cannot see pictures.

With a date in mind, we turned to practicalities. For us, this meant making a financial plan for the next year or two, deciding if we wanted to buy a house the next summer when our lease was up, switching to an insurance plan that covered pre- and postnatal care, and finding an ob-gyn so I could get a checkup and begin prenatal care. Fun stuff, huh? These topics ended up being good for us to address anyway, whether or not we were imminently becoming parents. Having a plan for these things helped shrink the list of "things I have no plan for or control over," which lowered my stress around being pregnant and having a kid. Looking back, we're grateful we had these conversations then as opposed to tackling them post-baby, when we were so sleep deprived we wanted to die.

Ready or Not

As you think about when and how to begin the journey toward parenthood, there are various factors to consider. You'll want to gauge how "ready" you feel, explore what methods are available for you to become parents, and examine the financial costs of adding a child to your family. If you are planning to pursue pregnancy, you might explore each of your medical histories and current health—as well as talk with your family members about their fertility experiences—to get an idea of how these factors might affect your overall timing.

It's also a good idea to look ahead to any big transitions on the horizon. Are you planning to move? Change jobs? Having a child is a huge change and combining it with another one will likely make it more stressful. Can you space out those events so you aren't going through them all at once? There may be a lot to this conversation, depending on your medical history, family-building plans, etc. I'd also like to point out there is a difference between being what I would call "logistically ready" and being "emotionally ready." Logistically ready is having the practical things lined up. Emotionally ready is feeling confident and at peace with your decision to become a parent. Personally, I was more logistically prepared than emotionally ready. But that's where knowing yourself is key. I knew I would never be fully emotionally ready to become a parent, but even so I wanted to be one. If I waited to feel emotionally ready, I never would have done it. All journeys to parenthood have their own beginning point, whether you choose pregnancy, surrogacy, adoption, or another method of building a family. I do want to stress that you should do what works for you as a couple, and you both need to be on board with the plan.

Finances

Finances are another aspect that may influence your timing. Most parenting experts agree that finances are one of the most important topics to address in your pre-kid discussions. The reason is twofold. First, money is the number-one source of conflict for couples; second, kids are hella expensive, and you are about to go through a significant financial transition in addition to a huge life transition. According to the renowned relationship scientists Drs. John and Julie Gottman in their book *Eight Dates: Essential Conversations for A Lifetime of Love,* statistics show that for a child born in the United States in 2015, it costs an average of $233,610 to raise that child through age seventeen. This includes things like food, healthcare, education, childcare, and clothing.[6] Multiply that amount by the number of children you want to have. And this is without factoring in any college expenses. Now, there's no need to start panicking because you don't have hundreds of thousands of dollars lying around, but you should take a look at how your finances will change after you have a child.

For many families, childcare is the biggest financial burden incurred after they have a kid. Keep in mind that the average cost for center-based childcare in the United States is $1,230 per month.[7] Take a look at options in your area or ask friends and family what their monthly budget for this is to get a sense of what you need to plan for. Remember, too, that there are many options when it comes to childcare, and everyone has a different situation. Again, do what works for you.

Depending on your path to parenthood, there may be an additional financial component to having a child. Medical bills from pregnancy and birth, adoption fees, sperm bank fees, or surrogacy payments are just some of the expenses you may incur. The reality for some couples is that you will need to assess whether you can afford to begin the process before you actually jump into it. This could mean researching the fees that might apply to your family. If you have insurance, what does it cover? What is the estimated out-of-pocket cost? Are there payment plans available? How might this fit into your budget?

I think the most useful, practical thing John and I did in this time period was meet with a financial advisor to discuss our long-term financial planning (that might be the most adult sentence ever). During our sessions we reviewed our current finances, discussed big purchases we planned to make in the next few years, reviewed our current retirement accounts and investment setups, made a plan for which debts to pay off in which order, and got recommendations for college funds for our future child. Our financial planner also laid out some long-term projections based on our income, investments, and anticipated retirement ages. It was comforting to see how certain decisions made now would lead to financial stability later on.

I struggle with financial discussions. About thirty seconds after someone says "taxes," their voice somehow changes into the one the teacher from the Charlie Brown TV specials uses, and I can no longer process any of their words. It wasn't realistic for me to do all that research and planning on my own, and John didn't want to take it on either. We thought of financial planning similarly to buying a house. Yeah, you *could* do it on your own, but it's a lot more work and you may or may not get it right. I suggest you hire a professional if you can afford it. It cost us about $1,500 up front but has undoubtedly saved us that and more over the years. Not to mention the time and energy saved not arguing about what to do with our money.

Whether you hire a professional or not, now is the time to hash out a budget. Don't wait until your child is three months old and you both need to go back to work and figure out childcare. If you keep separate finances from your partner and take turns with expenses, your shared costs will skyrocket when you have a kid. Making a plan for how to handle those together will save you arguing over whether your baby really needs new shoes, whose money to spend on music classes, or whether you can afford that fancy new crib. If this feels daunting, there are companies that specialize in helping couples hash out their finances. Try searching "financial coaching," and consider letting them be your guide. They charge less money than you would spend on a financial advisor, but they're still a knowledgeable, neutral party who can help you sort through those dollars and all of the emotions that come with them.

FINANCIAL CHECKLIST

- Compile your income and expenses and do the math to determine your current monthly budget (we use the software program You Need A Budget, and I highly recommend it).
- Decide if anything about your finances needs to logistically change; e.g., combining bank accounts, starting a new shared one, etc.
- Talk to your supervisor or human resources person at your workplaces to see what sort of leave is available and how it might affect you financially.
- Calculate potential childcare expenses for your area or look at how your income might change if one of you stops working. Ask friends with young children who live in your area or do some googling to figure out the numbers.
- Draft a new "after-kid" budget that includes the expenses you expect to have after you bring your baby home. Don't forget medical bills, large kid-related purchases like a crib or childproofing gear, diapers, formula, and a potential decrease in income if one or both of you takes a leave from work.

Even if you aren't in a place to make long-term financial plans, at minimum taking stock of your finances and making a short-term plan for how having a kid may affect them is helpful. In my family, where we both work full-time, we have a part-time nanny three days a week, John covers the other two, and I cover weekends when he works. Other families may do five days a week of daycare or school. Or they may have a parent stay home part-time or full-time. This is a personal decision based on your financial situation, desires for your child, and whether either of you has the preference or ability to stay home. The only thing I ask is that neither of you stay home because "it just doesn't make sense to work" or because "your salary would just be canceled out by the cost of daycare." If you want to work, work. If you want to stay home and you have that option, do it. But make it a choice. Don't let society or the patriarchy force you into it. The reality is that money is often tied up in power dynamics in life and in relationships, so you have to address those underlying dynamics as well as the practicalities of budgets, incomes, and spending.

Your Path to Parenthood

Let's take a look at the different options you can explore for becoming parents. Your path is going to directly affect your timing. Pregnancy takes at least ten months from conception, but this process can be delayed if conception doesn't happen easily. Adoption can involve six months of paperwork once you start the process before you can be eligible for a match. Assisted reproduction methods like in vitro fertilization (IVF) can add months or even years to your timeline. Each process has its own trajectory, so be sure to plan ahead as you look at various options. At the risk of repeating myself, I am going to reiterate that if you choose pregnancy as your path (assuming it is physically possible), the spouse who carries the pregnancy needs to be fully on board with that commitment. If you are in a couple where either partner has the physical ability to be pregnant, you need to decide which partner will carry the pregnancy. Then you may look into what you might need to do to prepare for becoming pregnant. You can decide if you want to track ovulation cycles, be on message boards, get an app, or, if you are a different-sex couple, just have a lot of unprotected sex and see how it goes. If you want to be really prepared, you can start looking into healthcare providers and decide if you want to work with an ob-gyn, a family doctor, or a midwife, etc. You and your partner should also discuss if you plan to tell people you are trying to get pregnant and how to handle questions if people ask. Before John and I began, I decided to get an ob-gyn checkup to make sure I was in good health and ask questions about trying to conceive, which made me feel more confident about trying to get pregnant.

Now, let's look at adoption. First, you need to decide what type of adoption you are interested in. Generally, there are three types: adopting a newborn, adopting from foster care, and adopting internationally. The timing for each is dependent on many factors, such as how fast you can do paperwork, if an expectant mother chooses you, travel requirements, cost, etc. Here's a breakdown of each in general terms:

- Adopting a newborn from the United States usually involves being chosen by an expectant mother who is making an adoption plan for her child. Assuming she continues with that plan after the baby is born, you might take the baby home within a few days to a couple of months, depending on the legal requirements in your area. You will likely have some sort of ongoing relationship with your child's birth mother, agreeing ahead of time to an open, semi-open, or closed adoption.

- Adopting from foster care can mean being a foster parent first, depending on your state, and may or may not involve the child's biological parents as part of the process. In Texas and possibly elsewhere, it's less likely that you will adopt a baby from the state unless they are part of a larger sibling group. This differs state by state, so you will want to explore your specific requirements.

• Adopting internationally rarely involves a child's biological parents, and these children are usually in either foster care or an orphanage setting. It typically requires traveling to another country for the legal process and to take placement of your child. The age range of children tends to be older, or children may have medical needs. This varies from country to country. Due to increased regulations and countries' desires to keep their children in their country of birth, international adoption placements have decreased in recent years, and have shifted away from placing babies. The total number of international adoptions to the United States reported by the Department of State in 2019 was 2,971. In 2005, the total number was 22,735.[8]

Adoption can be extremely complicated; the summary above is a very simplified description of the various methods. It's important to know what type you are looking into, as each has different requirements. Most people do their adoption research online; you'll find some places to start in the Resources section at the back of the book.

Once you decide what type of adoption you are interested in, you should review the requirements to determine if you are eligible for that program. Some countries or states require couples to be legally married for a specific period of time before adopting or be within a particular age range. Some are not accepting of single parents or same-sex couples. Depending on your circumstances, you may want to review the requirements online first to narrow down your choices. It can be helpful to look up general steps in the adoption process, so you know what to expect, and do research on agencies or lawyers to decide what avenue you want to pursue.

I am biased toward working with an adoption agency. Not only has this been my professional experience, but agencies are held to specific legal and ethical standards and often have processes in place to uphold those standards. They provide guidance on the process and emotional support for all of the parties involved. They act as a go-between when things get difficult or messy, and it's likely that at some point they will, since humans are messy. If you want someone to hold your hand through all of the stages of the adoption process, look for an agency. If you want to do most of that emotional and practical work on your own and just have someone take care of the legal side, look for a lawyer. It's difficult to know the timing with an adoption because each situation is unique, but a lawyer or agency should be able to give you an estimate so you can plan for that. While pregnancy and adoption are the two paths to parenting that I am most familiar with, there are of course other options, such as using a sperm donor, surrogacy, embryo adoption, or in vitro fertilization. They all have different processes, costs, and timing. Look into what might be a good fit for you as a couple based on your specific circumstances. (See the Resources section for more information.)

Whichever path to parenthood you choose, another decision to consider is if you plan to tell your friends and family that you are trying to start a family. I had read enough articles and blog posts about the annoyances of people constantly asking how getting pregnant was going to know I wanted to keep that information within the confines of our home. Luckily John agreed. We were fortunate that we didn't struggle with conceiving; if we had, I may have wanted to share that with certain loved ones in order to have more support. This may be different for you. Couples who are struggling with infertility might want to keep things to themselves, because it can be painful when others bring it up. I've also worked with adopting couples who wait to share with family until later in the game to avoid the constant questions about when they may get a child. You also might want to talk about when and how you want to share the news that you are expecting a child. Before I got pregnant, I thought that I would wait to tell anyone until we were past the twelve-week mark because of the risk of miscarriage. I didn't want to make big announcements and then have to go back and "untell" people if it didn't work out. In reality, when I got pregnant, I was bursting to tell people. I decided to share with those who would support us if a miscarriage occurred, and that decision felt right for me. There isn't a one-size-fits-all approach to building a family or the journey to getting there, so it is important to do what is right for you.

What Other Parents Said

One of the questions I asked the parents I interviewed was "What do you wish you had known before you became a parent?" I wanted them to share with me the things that might have made them feel more ready going in. Remember: You may never feel fully emotionally ready, and that's okay. The truth about becoming a parent is you don't really know what it is like until you get there. This is my best attempt to give you the inside scoop from other parents. Here is what they said:

DON'T SWEAT THE SMALL STUFF

"You think that the big stuff matters the most, but when they are tiny, just holding and loving on them is so important, and you can do that even when you feel like you are failing at everything else."

"I wish I'd had a better understanding that a lot of the decisions I would make as a parent are gut decisions, and a lot of times your gut is guiding you in the right direction, and that is often better than what society is telling you to do. I went in thinking breastfeeding was going to be a breeze, and it was not, and I felt a lot of guilt. Looking back, I can see it was not that big of a deal."

"I wish I had known to give myself more grace. When we were potty training, I felt so defeated. I have higher expectations and feel like I am failing her because I go to work all day and come home, and I can't teach her all the things. Now I know she will learn all of the things she is supposed to learn at her own pace."

"We did a lot of planning and thinking ahead of time, almost to the detriment of it. I wish I had known that it would all work out okay. We spent years planning and now I wish I could go out and take advantage of the freedom I had back then."

EMOTIONAL ROLLER COASTER

"How much shame and guilt can come in small moments as a parent. I was very hard on myself about not being able to meet my child's needs, and his emotions feeling so big for me."

"I was really sick the entire time my first pregnancy and that was hard. I didn't know it could happen. Also, while I felt

connected to the baby, my husband didn't really feel connected until our son was born, which was kind of hard."

"I wish someone had explained how you are going to change. The books tell you so much and it doesn't really feel personal. I wish people would talk about the emotions you go through. Our first was not planned, and my husband and I were not married at the time. It was very stressful. It was a roller coaster."

"I wish I had worked on myself a whole lot more in terms of pinpointing issues with anxiety—paying attention to what I needed to be mentally well and prepared so I could more fully be what my children needed from the beginning."

"Nothing can prepare you for being a parent, and nothing can prepare you for that up-all-night complete and utter exhaustion combined with hormones and feelings of rage toward your partner because they aren't the one having to get up and feed the baby. I was not prepared for the helpless feelings you get in the middle of the night when you are by yourself."

DEALING WITH CHANGE

"I thought I knew so much about taking care of kids, but I didn't know anything at all. It is totally different when you are taking care of your own kids. I had this idea of who I thought I would be as a parent, and when it's your own child all of those things fly out the window."

"How my wife would change toward me after having a child. It was all about the baby, which I am sure is true in most cases, but it was hard for me to handle my love life changing after becoming a parent."

"I wish I had known how much your priorities change. Before we had kids, my priorities were my wife and things we wanted to

do. But once we had kids, we had to be much more selfless to be effective parents, and my wife and I had to come to terms with that. There's just so much less that's about you and the things you want to do."

"How to just separate my opinion from everybody else's opinion. I didn't know it was coming, and it's been a learning process for me to weigh it and decide for myself what the best thing is for my child and our family."

"Before I had a kid, I was kind of afraid of the whole process, like I was going to be overwhelmed. I had a couple of cats and it didn't go well. Then I had a daughter and fell in love and can't get enough of her. I wish I had known this connection would happen, because it would have taken a lot of the fear away."

"I wish we would have known how kids change the dynamics between us and our parents. It's exhausting going between the grandparents sometimes. Knowing ahead of time what their expectations were would have been a nice conversation to have."

I SIMPLY CANNOT DO IT ALONE

"I wish I had known how to ask for help. That has always been something I've had an issue with. And the physical toll of birth in those first few weeks and how dependent this person would be on me, how to ask for help for myself so I could be there for her."

"I wish someone would have told me how difficult the immediate transition is and that it's okay to ask for help. Both of us were up all night and very tired, and we were stubborn at first and didn't want to ask for help. We felt like as new parents we should be able to do that on our own."

IDENTITY SHIFT

"I wish I would have known how different I was going to be—not in a bad way, but just that I never am going to be who I was before I got pregnant. It is wonderful and good and hard and challenging, but it would have been good to have the ability to know that and not be afraid of that and not be afraid of what parenting does to you."

"I wish I had known how difficult it was going to be afterward, not just getting used to having a kid around but how your body would be "OMG, what did you just do to me?" It took a while to realize that this is just what life is like now and you won't be the same as you were pre-baby. I was super fit before pregnancy, and worked out all through, and it has taken a long time to get back to that place."

PRACTICAL PLANNING

"I wish I would have been more prepared in the sense of daycare and savings. I had envisioned my mom taking care of my son but that didn't work out. I also didn't really know the financial cost of clothes, toys, etc."

"I am very Type A, Enneagram 1. I did a ton of research prior to my child coming home. I think I was as prepared as I could possibly be without actually having a child."

"I wish I'd known myself better. I did not know that I was an introvert, and I'd always had enough me time to not feel rundown. Had I known that before, I would have been better at figuring out self-care type things that would work for me. I am still trying to trudge through that and figure out what I really need to refill my cup and be the best provider for my child."

———

The through line for almost all of the responses from parents was that they didn't fully know the extent of how things would change when they had a kid. Whether we're talking about relationship dynamics or daily schedules or job fluctuations or changes in emotional health, the universal truth of becoming a parent is that it brings nothing but change. Most of us usually have a lot of fear around change because it represents the unknown. (We'll chat much more about fear in the next chapter.)

A few parents expressed regrets about not taking better advantage of their kid-free years. This also might be something to discuss with your partner. Is there anything you want to get out of the way before you have kids? John and I took a trip to Germany to tour the cities and visit the Christmas markets before we started trying to get pregnant. We had been talking about the trip for a while and the timing worked out, plus I knew I wanted to be able to drink on our trip, so I didn't want to be pregnant. While you can of course travel and do all sorts of other things when you have kids, it does get more complicated with planning, finding childcare, or the expense of bringing your child or children with you.

I also heard from parents again and again that there was no way they could have been truly prepared for the transition. Although it may seem counter to the point of this entire book, I think this is an important thing to remember. For the most part, parenting is a "learn as you go" experience. You can do the work to be ready for that learning, but one of the greatest tools you can bring with you is flexibility. When we do home studies for adoptive families, we look for families who demonstrate flexibility and have a means of emotional support. If you set yourself up to have both of those things, you are going to be just fine. (We'll do a deep dive on support in chapter 9.)

Summary

- Once you've chosen a path to parenthood it's time to talk about the details of what that looks like for you.

- Decide what factors affect your timing. Is it age, health, the number of kids you want to have, finances, etc.?

- Research shows that finances are one of the most important topics to discuss and plan for at this stage. If you can, meet with a professional to make a financial plan. If that is not realistic, focus on taking stock of your current financial situation and discuss how having a child will affect that.

- Seriously, talk about finances. Childcare costs are a bitch. You can use the Economic Policy Institute's website to find specifics on childcare costs in your state. (See the Resources section of this book for details.)

- When having your conversations about finances, talk about the power dynamics and emotions beneath financial decisions as well as the practical things like income, budgets, and spending.

- Decide with your partner when you plan to tell your friends and family about your impending parenthood. This decision will be different for every couple, so choose what works for you. Who and when will you tell that you are trying to become parents, are pregnant, etc.?

continues ›

- Becoming a parent brings nothing but change to your freedoms, your relationship, your schedule, your emotions, and your time.

- Now is the time to tackle your pre-kids bucket list. Are there any trips or projects you want to cross off before becoming parents?

- It is impossible to be completely prepared for the transition of parenthood. In addition to support (see chapter 9), the best tools you can have in your toolbelt are flexibility, pre-planning, and the ability to discuss decisions with your partner.

Discussion Topics:
Timing

1. Do you feel logistically ready to become parents? Do you feel emotionally ready? Why or why not? Is there anything you need to do to feel more ready?

2. What path to parenthood will you choose as a family? (Adoption, pregnancy, surrogacy, IVF, etc.)

3. How do you expect having a child to affect your finances?

4. When do you plan to begin that journey?

5. What do you need to do in order to begin? (Research agencies, get a checkup, toss the birth control, etc.)

6. What are your feelings around beginning that process?

7. When will you tell friends and family about beginning the path to parenthood?

8. When will you share news about impending parenthood with friends and family?

9. Will you make a social media announcement, mail announcements, etc.?

10. Did any of the quotes from other parents in this chapter bring up worries or questions for you?

Nothing to Fear but Everything

"Don't Panic."

—THE HITCHHIKER'S GUIDE TO THE GALAXY

PARENTING COMES WITH a side serving of fear, whether you want it to or not. The worry starts before your kid is even born and tends to not stop . . . ever. What makes becoming a parent so scary? For one thing, it is an irreversible decision. Once you have a kid, they are yours forever and you are stuck with them. There are no take-backs. If you are planning to parent with a partner, there is an extra layer of commitment required. While marriage is a commitment, it's one most of us feel we can get out of if we *really* need to. After all, our generation grew up when divorced parents were a dime a dozen. Once you have a kid with that person though, you are going to be forever connected—in some capacity—through your child.

But the main reason I think becoming a parent feels so daunting and can bring up so many fears is that it represents the great unknown. You just don't know what it's going to be like until you get there. And let's face it, being a parent is a huge responsibility. Having a child is just like embarking on a brand-new relationship, except you're the adult in charge who is supposed to know how to keep everyone safe and raise a responsible, contributing member of society. Maybe you barely feel like an adult yourself, and now you are going to be trusted with this helpless creature's entire life? Yikes.

If I am being totally honest, I can admit that when John and I started down this path, I was terrified of being pregnant. The whole thing sounded awful to me. Morning sickness, body changes, insomnia, hair growth in weird areas . . . ick. I asked several of my friends and family what the positive aspects of pregnancy were, and without fail every one of them said, "Well, you get a baby at the end"—and *that's it.* Seriously? Based on that information, I viewed pregnancy as more of a necessary evil or a means to an end. Now, having been through it, I can say it was not as scary as I thought it would be (things usually aren't). From my perspective, the positive aspects of pregnancy are as follows: no periods; ability to choose comfort over style in clothing; people being impressed when you do the things you would normally do non-pregnant; more pedicures, because you can't do it on your own; *and* you get a baby at the end. Pregnancy itself was one of my big fears about becoming a parent, but I had others, too.

- My entire life would change. I really liked my pre-baby life, and I knew that children change the dynamic of your life irreversibly. Maybe I would love our life with children even more than our life before. Or maybe I would mourn that old life.
- I would either have to do all of the work of parenting or drag John to do half, which basically amounts to the same thing. This is a real fear that I continue to struggle with in my marriage. I have a constant push-pull of

wanting to be in control of most things and also wanting to have an egalitarian household. It is a balancing act that I am still navigating.

- I wouldn't be able to relinquish control enough to let my husband do his part of the parenting work (see comment above about control).
- My career would be put on the back burner because at this point in our lives I make less money than John and because I am the mom—a.k.a. the default parent.
- We would struggle a lot as new parents without the support of family nearby.
- John and I had not had enough time to ourselves before adding children to the mix.
- Pregnancy and birth would be terrible, and all confidence in my body would disappear.
- We might not be able to become pregnant.
- Our baby might not be very cute. I know this is super shallow, but babies in my family are *gorgeous*. It's a lot to live up to. (Spoiler: they're adorable.)
- We were making a huge, life-altering decision that could turn out to be a mistake—and there was no going back.
- John might make a lot of promises about what type of parent he would be and then not follow through on them.
- We might screw up our kid.

Because I am an over-preparer, I signed John and me up for a "Bringing Baby Home" class offered at a local hospital. The class is part of the training curriculum designed by the Gottman Institute, and it covers the transition to parenthood and explores changes in your relationship that result. We were the only couple in the room who was not pregnant. As part of the training, they divided us into groups of men and women (all of the couples in our class were different-sex) to talk about our fears. I was feeling pretty good about myself because we had already done this at home, so I settled in to mostly listen and observe. Afterward, I asked John what fears the men talked about, and he said things like "that my wife will die during birth." Holy shit. That thought had never even crossed my mind! This was a good reality check for me. Here I was worried about how cute our baby might be, and other people were carrying around much more intense concerns.

Facing the Fear

I realize some of my fears may be shared by others, a few may be specific to me, and some are just wildly out of proportion. I made my list of fears in a fit of emotion one night when I felt like the whole world was on my shoulders. It had been sitting in my journal for a few months and I knew it was a discussion John and I would have to tackle. I also knew it would be a hard conversation, so I avoided it for a while. As with most situations, the hard conversations are sometimes the ones that need to happen the most. So when we finally set aside an evening to talk, I loaded up with a glass of wine and pulled out my list. John was unfazed that I had a list; in fact, I think he said something along the lines of "go ahead and get the list, I know you have one somewhere . . ." Points to him for knowing me. We dove in, and I lasted about five minutes before the tears came (what is it about getting older and crying? I find this has gotten much more frequent. And don't even get me started about post-pregnancy crying!).

The biggest fear we talked about was my concern that all of the parenting responsibilities would fall to me. This is not a new topic for us. We've had several conversations since we began dating about shared labor and being a team, and it's just an issue we'll likely have to manage throughout our marriage. As I struggled to explain to John why him forgetting to make dinner one night sends me down a spiraling black hole of anxious thoughts that end with him forgetting our children at the grocery store, and how that worry is linked to the concern that I will be a crazy control freak parent and not let him do anything, he dropped a truth bomb on me. It went something like this: "So you want me to be able to pull my half of the weight, and you are worried I won't, but at the same time you are also worried that you won't let me?" "Exactly!" I said, impressed by all he had surmised from my tear-choked rambling. Then he continued with, "Well, you know that will probably happen, because you can't just see a problem and not think of a solution for it, and immediately fix it."

Future-casting

This is how fear functions. Our brains are wired to make sense of things, and when we are faced with an unknown, they tend to fill in the blanks with whatever they can—often the worst-case scenario. Think about the last time your partner was late coming home from work and you called them and they didn't answer. You assumed they were dead, right? Or the last time you were walking through a dark parking lot alone, fighting off thoughts that someone was going to pop out and murder you. Our brains are wired first and foremost for survival. And that primitive part of our brain equates unknown with danger.

Here's how my brain works. John forgets to cook dinner one night. He has to scramble to come up with a last-minute plan to feed us. And *bam!* My anxious thoughts kick in. If he can't manage to feed two grown adults, how can he feed a baby? What if he forgets to feed the baby? What if he forgets the baby itself somewhere? Am I going to be the only one who is paying attention to this when we have a kid? And what about all of the other things you have to pay attention to? Will he even notice those things? Or will it all be up to me? Will I end up just having to do everything myself? I don't want to do that. But if I don't, will anyone else do it?

See how you can go down a rabbit hole? I remember having similar thoughts leading up to getting married. If John did some small thing that annoyed me, like smacking his gum, I would think, *Oh God, am I going to be able to tolerate this for the rest of my life? Am I really* choosing *to commit myself to this gum-smacker for better or for worse until death do us part?* This type of future-casting is totally fear-based, and often not rooted in reality. Let's look at the dinner example above. Yes, John didn't think about dinner ahead of time. Yes, he had to find a last-minute solution. But did we have dinner? Yes. He still met that need, albeit in a different way than I would have.

One way to process these kinds of situations is a trick I learned from Brené Brown, and it also helps when broaching fears with your partner. Take whatever you are thinking and put the phrase "The story I am telling myself is . . . " before it. As in "The story I am telling myself is that if John can't get dinner on the table until the last minute, I won't be able to trust that our children will be adequately fed." This does two things. It provides a reality check that just because you think it doesn't make it true. It's also a validation that this is a fear that you have, even though it's not necessarily a reality that is going to happen.

Now that we have two kids, I've realized that my fears around John not meeting their needs left out one key factor: Babies, and *definitely* toddlers, are pretty aggressive about getting their needs met. Although I don't think John would actually forget to feed our daughter, she's also going to announce loudly when she's hungry, and then have a total meltdown if someone doesn't get her food fast enough. That's a pretty big motivation for any parent. As time went on, I found that there wasn't as much on my shoulders to manage as I feared there would be when it came to day-to-day needs.

John and I discussed other concerns, such as my career being a priority, but also the reality that, from an economic standpoint, if one of us absolutely had to stay home, it would likely be me. I knew that I wanted to continue to work after we had kids, and I was worried that having a child would make me the default parent, and that this would affect my career growth. I was particularly sensitive about this topic since we had already moved to Houston for John's job. I felt like I had already sacrificed some career opportunity with that move, and adding kids seemed like a risk for more compromise. I wanted reassurance from John that he valued my career and would support me in it even after we had kids. He absolutely provided that for me. We also discussed that if we were to have a child with medical needs or that for some reason needed a full-time parent at home, that would likely be me, since the majority of our income came from John's job. I was okay with this hypothetical situation, and I figured we could work it out if and when that ever happened. For us, it was really helpful to talk about these issues. My feelings about maintaining my career have affected a lot of day-to-day parenting decisions, and being on the same page has helped eliminate what could have been a lot of conflict.

Another hot topic that brought on the tears was my concerns about how my body would change from pregnancy. I have basically had the same body since middle school, give or take some boobs. I've gotten really used to it and I like it. I feared the confidence I liked to think came from within was actually derived from the fact that I had society's preferred thin, small body type. And when that changed, what if I hated it? What if I got a belly where I didn't have one before? What if my boobs got saggy from pregnancy and breastfeeding? What if I ended up being a completely different size and had to buy all new clothes? What if pushing a baby out of my downstairs messed it up somehow and sex was ruined? Once these changes occurred, it seemed there was no going back. This is a hard topic for me to talk about, especially with other women. Full disclosure: I am a petite person; I wear size zero at most stores. I work out, but I eat pretty much whatever I want. I realize this is a blessing. I also have had enough women say something along the lines of "whatever, skinny bitch" that I know better than to bring it up. But it was there in the back of my mind when I thought about going through pregnancy and birth, and I knew my body would never be the same. Do you hate me yet?

John had many fewer fears than I did, and they were less detailed. He tends to go very logical with his worries, and also has the ability to *not worry about things that are out of his control*, which is basically magic to me. While I had worries about how cute our kids would be, he was afraid they might be dumb. My argument that one of those things is more fixable than the other was not well received. He also worried that he was going to be a "bad dad," but he couldn't really put into words what that label meant or what specifically he was afraid would happen. This was interesting to me. My first thought was that if he was sitting patiently on our couch while I sobbed into a glass of wine about how my boobs were going to look totally different and he better *get ready*, then he was going to be a pretty great dad.

I learned that John and I shared a few fears, too. The

main one was that we were going to do it all wrong and our kids would be totally screwed up. We might do something small when they were young that would traumatize them and stay with them forever. They might be dumb, and we would hold that against them. They might reflect the worst parts of ourselves, and it would be torture to see that come to life. They might hate us. We knew that we could read all the books and take all the classes and discuss things ad nauseam, but parenting is still basically a trial by fire. It's impossible to know how you will react to challenges in the moment. If we were lucky, we thought, we'd have years of trial and error to hopefully get it right.

Working with Fear

There's an episode of the television show *This Is Us* where the characters Randall and Beth, a married couple with three kids, are dealing with a potentially scary situation with one of their daughters. They play a game they call "worst-case scenario" where they list all of the terrible things they imagine could happen. They worry their daughter might become a stripper, rob them blind, or kill them both in their sleep.

Listing all the terrible thoughts swirling through your head may seem morbid, but it can also be freeing. The negative thoughts we have tend to wear us down when they stay trapped inside. When we share them, we lessen their power and split the burden. That's the goal here. Your fears may seem silly, or unrealistic. They might be things you have carried for years, or serious relationship issues that you need to go deeper on. Regardless, sharing them with your partner will allow them to know where you are coming from and will give you the gift of not being the only one to shoulder your worry.

The reality is that we all have fears, and whether they are logical, irrational, big, or small, they are *ours*. They are real and valid, no matter how insignificant or silly they may seem. Talking through your fears with your partner not only puts them out in the open, which in and of itself often makes them much less scary, but it also gives your partner clues about where you might need more support as you embark on this journey of parenting.

Bottom line: Speaking your fear out loud or writing it down takes away some of its power. Fear, like shame, grows in the dark and in secret. When I work with kids who've experienced trauma, a phrase we use often is "Name it to tame it." This means you need to get out in the open—to name—what is going on in your brain and body, which usually helps calm both down. John and I use it with our kids in naming feelings, but it also works for us.

A Word about Control

Whether you name them or share them, acknowledging your fears is key. In her book *Small Animals: Parenthood in the Age of Fear*, author and parent Kim Brooks writes:

> *Fear is neither wrong nor right. It is what it is. But in the end, it can't give us the things we most desire. It can't give us control. Nothing can. The control it offers is an illusion, a temporary distraction from the immutable fact that we're human, mortal, imperfect, and imperiled. There's no escape from that. Not for us and not for our kids. But when we accept it, there's a certain kind of freedom.*[9]

When we feel afraid, we want control. There are so many things we want to control when it comes to parenting, starting with conception, pregnancy, and birth. Control makes us feel safer, like the world is more predictable, and if we can figure out the system bad things won't happen. But no amount of control can actually guarantee challenges won't occur. Is it perhaps better to trade the illusion of control for the more vulnerable and scary feeling of freedom? Freedom to take things as they come, one day at a time. Freedom to figure problems out as they arise. Freedom to not have a plan for my child's entire life. I'm still working on letting go of some of that need to control and allowing myself the vulnerability to just be present. It sure sounds good, doesn't it?

Author Elizabeth Gilbert writes elegantly about fear in her book *Big Magic: Creative Living Beyond Fear*. The focus of the book is creativity, which I think is absolutely relevant here because I consider parenting the biggest creative challenge most of us will tackle in our lifetimes. Children are constantly growing and changing, and the moment you figure them out, they change again, and you have to start the creative process all over. Gilbert says, "Your fear will always be triggered by your creativity, because creativity asks you to enter into realms of uncertain outcome, and fear *hates* uncertain outcome."[10] That's it in a nutshell. We fear what we don't know. And when it comes to being first-time parents, there is *so much* we don't know, and won't know until we are in it.

Fear plays an important role in our lives as humans. Its job is to spot things that might be dangerous or harmful in order to help us stay alive and survive. But often it is set off by things that aren't actually threatening. In her book, Gilbert recommends having a little sit-down with fear. This is what we in the South like to call a "come-to-Jesus meeting." Gilbert starts her sit-down like this: "Dearest Fear: Creativity and I are about to go on a road trip together. I understand that you'll be joining us, because you always do." She goes on to tell fear that although she knows it is along for the ride, it won't be allowed to drive.[11] This is obviously metaphorical and might seem a little silly, but again, speaking things out loud often makes them less scary. Fear can be respected and acknowledged and at the same time not be allowed to overtake your life. This is a good thing to start practicing now. Let me tell you, the fears tend to increase once your kid arrives.

What Other Parents Said

When I talked with other parents, I found that most of their fears fell into three categories: pregnancy and birth, keeping a tiny human alive, and not fucking up your kid.

PREGNANCY AND BIRTH

"Once I was pregnant, I was like, 'Oh shit, I have to push this baby out of me.' The unknown of birth was scary. You can read about it, but you don't really know. The second and third time I wasn't worried about it at all."

"I was afraid I wouldn't be able to get pregnant, and in fact, it took four years and more money than we had. My anxiety became intense and focused during pregnancy. I was afraid of losing the baby. I was afraid of something happening to me or the baby or both and leaving my husband alone. I was afraid of an emergency C-section. I was afraid of birth defects or injury. Once I could feel the baby moving around, it helped calm some of my fears because I could tell she was alive and healthy. My fears were very much focused on pregnancy and birth. I wasn't really afraid of becoming a parent at all."

"What if our baby is born with a third arm? And other irrational fears."

"Not knowing when I was going to go into labor made me anxious, just not knowing what it felt like and when it would happen. I was also worried about having an emergency C-section."

"Birth and recovery. I didn't know the nitty-gritty of it, and it kept me up at night. I also worried about breastfeeding."

"I was afraid of losing the pregnancy, and fearful of something happening to the baby or my wife during childbirth."

"Prior to getting pregnant, my biggest fear was not being able to conceive. Once we accomplished that my fears shifted to maintaining a tiny human life."

"I was terrified that pregnancy might be terrible, and all of the physical repercussions of birth. It ended up being honestly easy for me."

"My first pregnancy was scary the whole time because I didn't know if I would be able to carry it to term. I also had insulin-dependent gestational diabetes, so I worried about if he would be healthy."

"I had a friend who had a late-term miscarriage, so the whole time it was hard for me to be excited because I was worried that would happen. And then I fell on my stomach a week before my due date, and that was scary, but everything was fine. It was hard to set up the nursery, etc., because I didn't want to do all of this and have my heart broken. I also had fear that there would be some medical needs."

KEEPING A TINY HUMAN ALIVE

"I worried about having a healthy baby and things going well. I was worried about if we would have a good support system because none of our families were nearby."

"The first three months were just . . . is he going to die in the crib?"

"How to handle two babies at once! Twins have a way of making you accept things as they are and let go a little because you just can't control everything."

"I was anxious about SIDS (sudden infant death syndrome) and control. Something could happen and I would have absolutely no control over it and that was terrifying. I was also fearful of choking, and I still have that fear. I obsess over him chewing food, size of bites, etc."

"Keeping a human alive. I was never into holding anyone's baby; they seemed so fragile. Our child was the first I ever held that young. Once they got past age two, I felt a little better. I didn't want anything to happen to them, everything that had to do with keeping them safe. Every sound they make early on you think they are dying."

"The hospital scares the shit out of you about SIDS."

"I was anxious about all of the little tasks I was going to learn how to do and I didn't want to screw them up. I had never held a newborn baby before mine was born, so I had to learn all the basics of how to keep them safe and alive."

NOT FUCKING UP YOUR KID

"I don't know if I feared being a bad parent before I had kids. I thought I knew what I was doing. Now I fear being a bad parent."

"I worried about not being good enough and not being able to provide."

"I was afraid that I'd mess it up. Like, long-term mess it up. I still have that fear a little bit. I think about things we do now and if they will bite us in the butt down the road."

"I was afraid of doing something that would damage her long-term. I had a complicated childhood, so my fear was, How will I protect her from some of the things that I went through. Not knowing if I am doing everything right and if I will be able to keep her safe."

"The pressure of helping them be all that God has created them to be, and the responsibility of all we have to teach them as parents."

"I was—and still am—terrified of those moments where I imitate some of the more hurtful behavior I received from and saw modeled by my own father. I would say all of my fear pre-parenting was wrapped up in this idea—scared that my kids wouldn't get the kind of love they needed from me."

Motivating Fear

I think many parents worry about the same things, but since we don't typically talk about fear, we often feel like we are the only ones to experience it. It doesn't help that most of us might not feel safe talking with others about our feelings around trying to have a kid, because we don't want to endure the constant questions about how it's going or when we are going to have a baby already. I hope that reading these thoughts from parents helps you feel less alone in your journey. Unfortunately, fear can contribute to making early parenthood a lonely time, which is why it is so helpful to find other parents in the same stage as you (more on that later.) But remember: fear is natural, especially as we head into the unknown. For a lot of us, parenting is the biggest unknown we have tackled in our lives.

I'd almost be concerned if you *didn't* have any fears going into parenting, as sometimes those fears actually serve a purpose. Kim Brooks introduces the concept of motivating fear in her book *Small Animals*: "I've come to think of one strain of this fear as *motivating fear*, and it is a form of anxiety that was intensely familiar to me from the moment I learned I was pregnant. Motivating fear is fear that compels a parent to do something for or with or on behalf of her child."[12] This concept resonated with me. As I read through the thoughts other parents shared, so many of them seemed to have a motivating factor. The father who felt unloved by his own dad and wants his child never to feel that way. The many parents who gave their actions so much weight that they felt that one slip-up could ruin their child for life. The parents who felt a higher power had designed their child to be something great, and that they were responsible for developing that greatness. All of these parents are extremely motivated to do their best every day, to make sure their child knows they are loved, and to parent with intention and deliberation.

Let's look at the difference between unhelpful fear and motivating fear. Unhelpful fears are vague, absolute, and usually exaggerated. Motivating fears are concrete, feelings-based, and actionable. Here are some examples:

Unhelpful Fear	Motivating Fear
"I might totally fuck up my kid because I don't know what I am doing."	"I am new to this job of parenting and it feels huge and overwhelming."
"My partner might not do as much work as I will, and all of the parenting stuff will fall on me."	"How my child is cared for is very important to me and I want to make sure that they are safe and content."
"My parents did something hurtful to me, and I might do the same thing to my child."	"Being aware of how I was hurt as a child will help me to parent in a different way."
"The decision I make now might totally mess something up down the road."	"The best I can do is to make thoughtful and informed decisions with the information I have in the moment."

Try this exercise. Write down your most dramatic fear. Now look at what drives it. Say you wrote down "I am going to be a bad parent." What's really beneath that fear? Is it that you have zero experience with children? Is it that your parents weren't great role models, and you are afraid you will be like them? Do you have a very demanding job and worry you won't be around as much as your kid might need? See if you can name your fear to tame it, and turn it into a concrete, feelings-based thought. This will make your worry easier to tackle. For example, you can learn more about children if your experience is limited. You can work with a therapist to process hard experiences from your childhood. You can weigh your career and home priorities and make changes if you need to. If you dig a little deeper, not only can you ease some of the fears, but you may also be able to make them work for you. As a final thought, I encourage you to see your fears not merely as an enemy you must overcome, but also, sometimes, as the push you need to be the best parent you can be. Bring fear along for the ride. It's not going anywhere, but you don't have to let it drive.

Summary

- Grabbing a glass of wine, a chocolate bar, or your vice of choice and sitting down with your partner to name all of your fears about parenting can be a very bonding and freeing experience.

- Your fears are valid, no matter how big or small, realistic or imagined.

continues ›

- Many parents-to-be have similar fears. Those expressed by the parents I interviewed broke down into a few categories, namely pregnancy and birth, keeping a tiny human alive, and not fucking up your kid.

- Fear can be scary, but when framed correctly, can also motivate you to be a better parent.

Discussion Topics:
Fears

1. Exercise: Write a list of all of your fears about parenting and share them with your partner.

2. Pick your greatest fear and tell them why it looms so large.

3. Talk about how you can help each other manage your fears as you go through this process.

4. Write your own letter to fear telling it that you recognize its purpose, but it is not in charge. Start with "Dear Fear . . ."

5. Think about how your fears could motivate you as a parent.

Hopes, Dreams, and Expectations

*"Hope is being able to see that there
is light despite all of the darkness."*

—DESMOND TUTU

NOW THAT I have sent us all down an anxiety spiral about all of the things that could go wrong when it comes to being parents, let's bring the mood up a bit. Despite my many fears and worries, the driving factors in my desire to become a parent were my hopes and dreams. I had several things I was looking forward to with my future children and family. I knew some of these expectations would be realistic, and some might not. Nonetheless, they were fun to talk about, to dream about, and to share with others. Here are some of the things I anticipated:

- My children having success in their lives, whatever that looks like for them.
- I hoped parenting would bring a new layer to the team of my marriage, and I looked forward to seeing my husband as a dad.

- I think children are hilarious, and I looked forward to all of the ways we would laugh together.
- I looked forward to seeing all of our parents be grand-parents (they are going to rock it).
- I hoped my children would have connections with cousins, aunts, and uncles, as I did.
- I couldn't wait to see the world through the eyes of my child.

What I never could have anticipated—or prepared for—is the rush of love I felt after my daughter was born. I don't recall exactly when it happened, maybe later that day, maybe in the next couple of days. I was pretty tired and foggy from forty hours of labor and pushing a human out of my body. But that rush of love? It hit me hard. It was like nothing I had ever felt before, and it was wonderfully overwhelming. Remember when you were in high school and you fell desperately in love with someone? You became completely obsessed with them, memorized their schedule, doodled in notebooks about them, and thought about them all the time. You daydreamed about what they were doing when you weren't together, and even when you spent every waking hour with them, a few minutes away left you missing them, and feeling as if there were a hole in your world. That's what it feels like when you fall in love with your tiny human. If anyone had tried to tell me what it would feel like beforehand, I would not have been able to grasp it merely from words. I had to go through it to be able to experience the magic that is the deep, unshakable love you feel for your child.

Now that I am in the thick of parenting, I have seen a lot of my expectations realized and experienced joys I never could have foreseen. Please allow me to be that cheesy "being a parent is the most fulfilling thing" person for just a minute.

There are depths of emotion I have experienced as a parent that seemed to have been locked to me before. Hearing my husband making our toddler giggle uncontrollably, or telling her "I know, it's so hard" when she is upset. Seeing the unabashed love and mutual obsession between our daughter and her grandmothers. Getting tiny hugs and slobbery kisses. I am actually tearing up as I write this. I didn't know how these things would feel until they happened. They are delightfully, incredibly joyful and touching. Have you ever had that feeling where something is so beautiful or wonderful that it takes over your body and you just have to cry, because you have to let such a strong feeling out? Perhaps you felt it while looking at a glorious aspect of nature, like the ocean, or finding a piece of art that was unbelievably beautiful to you. Remember that feeling? It's that, times ten. I used to think people who cried from happiness were ridiculous. Now I am pretty sure they are all just parents.

That said, I do want to honor those who may be reading this and can think of absolutely nothing they are looking forward to about being a parent. Maybe you've never really spent time with children, so you only know the stories people tell you. Why is it that all of the people you know feel the need to tell you their horror stories when they find out you are having a kid? Yikes! Let's spread some light, people. Maybe you are so full of worry and anxiety about those intense early days of trying to survive and keep this other human alive that you just can't get past it to thinking about what good stuff may be coming. I see you. That's perfectly okay, and also pretty normal. Don't beat yourself up if you don't have a list of joys you are looking forward to about being a parent. These can also be vague and abstract, such as "I hope my child is happy with their life," or "I hope they contribute to society." And don't get down on your partner if they can't come up with anything, even if you happen to have a list a mile long. It's okay for you to be in different emotional spaces about this huge life change.

If you are having trouble coming up with an entire list of things to look forward to, try to pick just one. Are you excited about seeing this person you love and chose to partner with in life evolve alongside you? Are you curious about who your child will grow up to be? Are you picturing yourself snuggling a warm baby as they drift off to sleep, content in your arms? Can you envision holding the chubby hand of your toddler as you take a walk, stopping to exclaim over a leaf, a caterpillar? Pick one thing to hold on to, big or small. Because the joyful stuff will come. You will have a tiny hand grab your finger, or a toddler squeal with delight and run to greet you when you come home from work, and you'll think, *There it is.* Be gentle with yourself. Give it time.

If you truly have no idea what having a baby will be like, find someone who does and ask them to be honest with you about the good and the bad. This might be your mom, dad, aunt, uncle, friend, coworker, cousin, brother, or sister. Or even an online group full of strangers. Most parents are willing to tell their story and share their experience. My hope is that we have evolved from the days when we had to look like we had it all together. We seem to have accepted, on some level, that we are all in this big, beautiful mess as humans together, and we need to do what we can to help each other out.

Once you've identified those things you are looking forward to (even if it's just one), talk about those hopes and expectations together. Hearing about your partner's expectations can help you learn more about them. Perhaps they dream of a daughter to play dress-up with, or a son to obsess over sports with. Exploring expectations about parenting with your partner can help you go into this huge life change with your eyes wide open—and avoid surprises or conflicts down the road. Remember the first thing on my list? *I hope my children have success in their lives, whatever that looks like for them.* For John and me, this sparked a conversation about how I defined success, and if that meant I expected all of our children to go to college. It was an important conversation to have in terms of planning for the future. Let's say I defined success as getting a college degree. That would affect my parenting for most of my child's educational journey. It might influence where we live if being in a "good" school district was important to us, or lead me to push my child to be in more academic-focused activities rather than arts or sports. It might create an undercurrent of pressure for my child to perform that would only let up when they walked across the stage on graduation day. As John and I talked about this, we agreed that we didn't automatically expect our children to go to college unless it was a good fit for them. We expected them to be responsible, to grow to be independent and self-sufficient, and to explore things they were passionate about.

Now, the caveat to having expectations is to keep them in check. While dreams are lovely, as parents we can't always control what our children end up being passionate about. I probably don't have to tell you this, but research shows that unrealistic expectations can be a risk factor for developing postpartum mood and anxiety disorders, often referred to as PMADs (along with other environmental factors, genetic history, and hormonal fluctuations).[13] What if you get a daughter who hates to dress up? Or a son who is more into art than football? How would you handle that? I think most of us don't go into parenting planning to be *that person* who lives vicariously through their child, but those expectations can get in the way sometimes. It is a lot easier to avoid this if you are aware of what they are, and how they might affect you.

Here's an example. When we were deciding on names for our daughter, I was adamant about choosing one that would result in her being taken seriously when she grows up, as this was an expectation I had for her. I had certain names that I felt might hold her back in the world as a woman, and I wanted to avoid them. If you haven't noticed, names have gotten pretty creative in the United States lately. When I was pregnant, I read somewhere about doing the "Supreme Court Justice" test for names to meet this qualification. Here's how you do it. You take your baby's name and put "Supreme Court Justice" in front of it. If it doesn't sound plausible, you toss it. For example, Supreme Court Justice Toots McGiggles is just not going to be a thing. I put a lot of stock in this, and honestly, I still kind of do. Women have enough barriers to overcome without being discounted because of a ridiculous-sounding name. And that doesn't even begin to scratch the surface of the judgment and discrimination people with "non-White"-sounding names face. But honestly? My daughter is going to make her way in the world no matter her name, and I probably overanalyzed it. And no, we did not name her Ruth Bader Ginsburg—although I wasn't opposed to it.

What Other Parents Said

In my interviews with parents, I asked them to share what they looked forward to before becoming a parent. There were so many sweet answers—from daily rituals like reading together to watching them learn and discover to finding the kid in yourself again. See if some of these resonate for you.

RITUALS AND TRADITIONS

"I looked forward to holidays, because that was a big thing in my childhood. My mom made all of the holidays super special, even on Flag Day, when we would make our own flag."

"Christmas morning, and other things that were meaningful to me from my childhood. I envisioned him running down the hallway at our house giggling. With adoption there is hesitancy to get attached to a certain idea, so we had to hold ourselves back on that a little bit."

RAISING GOOD PEOPLE

"I hoped that my kids would be healthy and happy. And that they would make better decisions than I did as an adolescent."

"I hoped that we would raise good kids who would become good adults."

"I hope that my kids are good, passionate, purposeful."

"I want my kids to be kind and caring for others and to themselves."

"I want my kid to grow up to be a kind, responsible, good human. I want him to know he has a team behind him to support him. I want him to have a family."

"My greatest hopes were and are simply that my children would have good health and will be kind to others."

KNOWING THIS NEW PERSON

"As a biracial couple I was very excited about seeing what our kids would look like."

"I looked forward to holding the baby, seeing what they looked like. Seeing their personalities grow, talking with them, and telling them stories."

"I'm looking forward to knowing him and getting to experience small and big moments with him."

"Seeing this blob turn into a person and what she would be like. Watching her grow. And who we would become as a family and as parents."

"I pictured having a rocking chair and sitting there reading a book to my son. Seeing me and my child, what they would look like, what their interests would be."

FAMILY CONNECTIONS

"I was excited for my parents to be grandparents again."

"I looked forward to having a fan. I was such a fan of my dad, and I was excited to have that relationship, and in return be their biggest fan."

"My dad and I didn't have the best relationship, and I like that I can be a father to her and be the things that I never had. I want her to grow up with a good idea of what men are."

"I was excited to have those family moments together and create moments for them to experience life together. Also, to have kids to invest in; I loved my family dynamic growing up, so I was looking forward to recreating that in our family."

"Bonding and attaching with her. Even now I look forward to the reaction I get when I walk through the door after being gone all day. The love that I can tell that she knows I have for her and how she reciprocates that. I always wanted that, and I am so happy that we have it."

"I wanted to pass on a lot of what my parents did during my childhood, which was a special time for me. Looking forward to that family togetherness, which is why I wanted a big family, and I wanted my kids to have siblings."

"I wanted to see what he would look like or be like as a combination of us. We bought a house right before we started trying, so I would picture the nursery and a game room full of toys. A house full of noise and play. Sort of filling up everything in our lives."

"How it would bring my husband and me closer together and how we would grow, and then what our child would look like putting our genes together. Doing the things we liked to do, traveling, hiking, etc., with our child."

KID ACTIVITIES

"I always knew I was going to be a boy mom, so I was looking forward to going to sporting events, being active, having 'mama's boys.'"

"I was excited for him to play sports, play outside, go fishing, and to teach him things."

"Tucking a kid in at night; my parents would tuck us in at night and talk about the day together. I like reading to my daughter every night now, and we get to lay in the bed and read a book and snuggle."

"I'm looking forward to going hunting with my kids and my whole family."

EXCUSE TO BE A KID AGAIN

"Doing all the things that you don't have justification to do as an adult, like going to parks, museums, etc. Showing her all the places that are special to us and seeing her reaction."

"Playing. I heard that you get to rediscover everything that your kid is going through for the first time and thought that would be fun. Like if they are super into bugs, or whatever they get into. You get to kind of be a kid again. With a kid everything is new and different. She doesn't have any 'life filters' on yet. You get to see the small details around you that you don't really notice."

"It's a good excuse to go to toy stores. Take her to baseball games. Try to get her to like all the stuff that you like."

Second Chances

You may have noticed a few statements from parents that expressed a desire to create the type of relationship they never had with their parents, sort of like a "do-over" for that parental connection they wish they'd had. If this is you, explore that, possibly with a therapist. Although it is a lovely sentiment to want to create a strong, positive relationship with your child, if you are saddling them with the pressure of giving you that connection you felt was missing with your own parents, it may backfire on you. It is our responsibility as parents to be emotionally attuned to and care for our children, not the other way around. Making your child responsible for your emotions gives them a lot of power over you and sets them up for potential struggles down the road. We will explore this issue further in our discussion of attachment theory in chapter 6. For now, this is just a word of caution, in case you find yourself going there.

Summary

- Sharing the hopes you have for your children tells your partner what you are looking forward to about being a parent and gives you both an opportunity to explore expectations about your future child.

- It is perfectly normal to have a hard time coming up with things you are looking forward to about having a kid. If this is you or your partner, be gentle with yourselves, and maybe try to find one simple good thing to look forward to.

- Exploring expectations can help us check to see if they are realistic and allows us to go into situations with our eyes wide open.

- Unrealistic expectations can be a risk factor for developing postpartum mood disorders.

Discussion Topics:
Hopes

1. Talk about, and perhaps make a list, of the "big-picture" things you look forward to or expect from your future child or children. Do you envision them playing sports? Being an artist? Advocating for climate change? Do you want them to be brave, sensitive, kind?

2. Now make a list of the small joyful moments you are looking forward to, like baby smiles, laughter, playing at the park together, baking cookies, holidays.

3. Choose one thing that you love about children and talk about how you may experience that in parenting.

4. What are your dreams for your future family? If you imagine yourself twenty years into the future, what does that look like?

5. How might your expectations affect how you parent? Are your expectations realistic? Flexible? Check to see if your expectations are more about you, or about your child.

Ch-Ch-Ch-Changes:
Dealing with Transition

*"The biggest thing I remember is
that there was just no transition.
You hit the ground diapering."*

—PAUL REISER

TRANSITIONING TO PARENTHOOD is a major shift that brings many changes. Most parents can't fully appreciate this until it happens, but there are ways to set yourself up for success. In this chapter, we're going to focus primarily on how having a child may alter your relationship with your partner and look at strategies for maintaining connection.

What Other Parents Said

During my conversations with parents, I asked them to share how their relationship with their spouse changed after they had a kid. Their responses were quite varied. Some experienced a level of intimacy in parenting that they had never known before. More than a few found having a kid exposed all of the vulnerabilities of the relationship. For some couples, one partner struggled with the transition more than the other. Almost every parent talked about having less time together as a couple. All of these are normal ways for your relationship to change after having a kid. Here's what they said:

KIDS COME FIRST

"We have both become much more focused on our child than on each other, but we are both in agreement that that's where we want our focus for now. She's still very young and needs a lot of attention, but we know that won't last forever. We definitely have much less time to do the kinds of things we used to do together, but we do a lot of fun things as a family now instead. We also have set date nights about once a month that allow us to get out together for at least a couple of hours."

"It has changed a whole lot. In the beginning it felt like my wife forgot about me. It was almost like we were just roommates after the baby was born. No affection/intimacy (nonsexual). My wife was focused on the baby."

"My husband would say that it changed completely. We didn't have an opportunity to be a married couple for very long before we got pregnant. Our whole marriage has been trying to figure out parenting together, and a lot of times our relationship takes a backseat to that."

TIME TOGETHER

"We are working on remembering that we were a couple before we were parents, but our relationship is sometimes nothing but household management for weeks at a time. At the same time, we have a connection that literally cannot be broken and a respect for each other as parents that can't come from any

other role in life. No matter what happens, I will always love and respect my partner as a father and that cannot be replaced."

"We don't have the same amount of time to do whatever we want to do. We still spend a lot of time together but it's mostly doing what the kids want to do. We have to communicate differently and make sure we are on the same page before we present things to the kids. It deepens your relationship because you are working on this big project together, and it also is sink or swim because if you aren't on the same page it drains your relationship. Also, as a woman your body completely changes and that changes the dynamic as well."

"At first my partner was amazing. He stepped up for a while and was really excited, and then it started to fade away. I think it put fear in him that his life was changing. If you're someone who avoids a lot of issues, it's going to be difficult because you have to come to terms with your life changing."

COMMUNICATION

"It made us communicate a lot more effectively. We learned so much more about how we perceive each other, how we approach each other, tone of voice, time of day, etc. It has given us a lot more respect for each other because you see each other really just stripped down to your most vulnerable, and there is so much strength to see in that, which we never would have seen if we didn't have kids. It's given us more purpose to how and why we invest in our marriage. And motivation to set aside time for each other and be intentional in that."

"It changed some things for the better. One of the things we struggled with as parents was that all of a sudden if I decided to do something it had a big effect on my wife. The amount of coordination that has to take place between the two of you increases tenfold. We had to learn how to really understand each other and communicate with each other better, and we have."

WORKING AS A TEAM

"I love my husband so much more than I ever knew I could. It has not been stressful in our marriage. We really feel like we are such equal partners and can tag in and out. I feel supported and loved by my husband in a deeper way, and I feel like we have been able to connect emotionally on a deeper level than before we had a kid."

"The transition was good and was challenging. We were in it as a team, and it was something we were doing together and figuring out together. The hard part was maternity leave with our first child, when I was alone with her a lot and he was working more. Bearing the brunt of childcare during that time was hard. We are still working on sharing childcare and chores."

"Obviously, there was more stress to navigate with the arrival of a kid, but I also think we bonded over how much we both wanted to be the best parents possible. Parenting brings out so many latent issues from one's own childhood that have gone unresolved, and, in some ways, we had to learn a new language in order to communicate with each other about the origin of things we were struggling with in our marriage or in our parenting. In many ways, identifying the baggage we bring with us has helped us be a better team—understanding each other's strengths and weaknesses."

"Pre-kid, we were free spirits. We could go out and do this or that, and not be as conscious about the other person's feelings. When you have a child, you are very sensitive to your partner's feelings because if you aren't it is going to be really hard to parent. We are a lot more mature just for the fact that we have to be. We recognize that she sees us and will mimic anything and everything. Having those little eyes constantly on us makes us much more conscious about how we interact with each other."

"We were together for eleven years before we had kids, so I feel like we make a pretty good team. Our tempers have gotten shorter with each other, but our patience has gotten better. We have gotten better at apologizing to one another when we get frustrated and it's been a long day. It's changed a lot, but it's also confirmed that my husband is the guy and the dad I thought he was going to be. We don't get to spend as much time one-on-one, but that relationship is still there."

NEW CONNECTIONS

"We had a healthy and established marriage prior to having our first daughter. I thought I knew what to expect from my husband. Wasn't that silly? In some ways, of course, adding a child was a difficult transition. The most incredible thing though is that I discovered a new love for my husband that I didn't know existed. I love him for myself and I now also love him as the father of my children. I would say it's a deeper, more comprehensive love that bonds us."

"I think it's really hard in the first part, right after they are born; there is so much that is on the mom. You're the feeding vessel; the baby is calmed by you; your reaction to crying is different. That was hard because I felt like I was doing everything, and I was very resentful. At the same time, there is nothing like seeing your spouse love your kid. My husband is a very stereotypical engineer—emotion is not his thing. I love seeing the way his heart has opened up with our son."

"It's important to be realistic, especially in the first year, and give your relationship some grace. There were times where I felt 'touched out' and could not take being touched by anyone else except the baby. My husband's primary love language is touch, and he felt rejected when I couldn't be touched. Counseling has deeply impacted how we relate to each other,

*and I feel grateful that we had that relationship established
before we had a kid."*

———

I think this paints a good picture of what the transition to
parenthood can look like when it comes to your relationship
with your partner. If reading through these comments made
you worried, I have good news: there are evidence-based
methods for safeguarding your relationship during this transition. We'll get into those later in the chapter; for now, I'd
like to share the story of my own transition journey.

What I Learned

Having a kid was one of the biggest changes in my life
and definitely the most unpredictable. I had given *a lot* of
thought to the fact that a baby would change everything
(hence the entire chapter on fears). One area that I particularly obsessed over was my marriage. I liked my pre-kid
relationship with John, and as we have already established,
for me change = anxiety and fear. I knew that having a baby/
toddler/preschooler would be hard, and that those years
would include stress, juggling, and much less sleep. I knew
the average length of a marriage that ends in divorce in the
United States is eight years, when many couples exit the
fog of baby- and toddlerhood and reassess their happiness
in their relationship.[14] This knowledge only fueled my worries. Talking these thoughts through with John helped me
bring all of my concerns out into the open as issues we could
tackle as a team rather than just things I ruminated on; it
also gave me at least a glimmer of control amid all the chaos
of the unknown. And talking about it with other expectant
parents helped me realize that I was not alone.

But talking wasn't enough. As is typical for me, I took to the internet to get some additional information to obsess over and analyze. As discussed earlier, I happened upon a class offered by the Gottman Institute called "Bringing Baby Home." John and Julie Gottman are the well-known scientists who developed an experiment in which they observe couples and can predict from their interactions whether they will stay together or get divorced, and whether they will be happy in their relationship. A scientifically proven way to safeguard my relationship? Sign me up!

Sign me up indeed. John pulled on his good-sport pants yet again and cheerfully (okay, resignedly) joined me for a weekend of fun (class). Taking this class made me feel like I was actually doing something to prepare, and since I'd been having trouble finding the parenting information I'd been looking for, it was nice to land there. In the class we covered topics like building connection with your partner, how to approach conflict and problem-solving, connecting with your child, and preserving intimacy and romance. There was a pretty heavy focus on couples having a biological child together, but my general experience with the Gottman Institute's work has given me the impression that they value inclusivity, and their strategies apply to all couples, so I would recommend it for any partners wanting to do a deeper dive into this piece of preparing for the parenting transition. (See the Resources section for more information.)

Time Shift

One of the major areas of focus for this class was the reality of how all-consuming it is to care for an infant. To drive this point home among the class participants, the facilitators had us do an exercise where we filled in a pie chart for time spent in all of the areas of our lives, and then talked about how we might fit it all in after we have a baby. My chart looked like this:

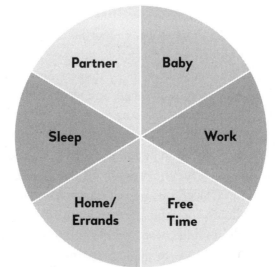

Realistically, it should have looked like this:

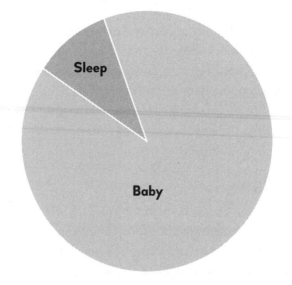

Seriously, ask anyone who has ever had a newborn. This is accurate. See how there's not a lot of time for anything? Even your partner? That can be a problem, especially if you fall into the habit of not making time for each other long after the days of the newborn fog have passed. While many new parents assume they will "get back to" finding a connection with their partner down the road, the Gottmans maintain the importance of actively prioritizing connection in your relationship early on.

Maintaining Connection

In their most recent book, *Eight Dates*, the Gottmans boil down the two things they recommend couples do to maintain satisfaction in their relationship through the transition of having children. First, they recommend that both partners be involved during pregnancy, birth, and with the new baby. This applies to both same-sex and different-sex couples, though their studies showed that in different-sex couples, dad's involvement takes on a greater significance (we'll talk more about this later in this chapter). Second, they say couples must make an effort to maintain intimacy and connection and prioritize their relationship.[15] This may seem impossible in those early days, but I promise it isn't. In a nutshell, the Gottmans' premise is that there are scientific behaviors that bond couples together, and also those that erode their connection. Here are a few of them:

BONDING BEHAVIORS

- Turning toward "bids for connection," such as when your partner shares happy news and you are happy with them.

- Supporting your partner when they are struggling or sad by listening, taking tasks off of their plate, giving them a hug, or giving them space.
- Responding positively to a touch or eye contact.
- Meeting a partner's need when they ask for something; for example, "Can I have a hug?"
- Doing something kind for your partner, like cooking them dinner or picking up their favorite snack at the store.
- Spending time with your partner being fully present.
- Holding your partner's hand if they reach for yours.

ERODING BEHAVIORS

- Ignoring your partner
- Rejecting attempts at connection
- Criticizing your partner
- Name-calling
- Blaming and shaming

One of the most important bonding behaviors is responding to "bids for connection," such as sharing happy or sad news or reaching to hold our partner's hand. When the bid is answered (our partner celebrates with us or accepts our invitation to hold hands) it builds our connective bond. John Gottman also talks about what he calls "the four horsemen of the apocalypse," a rather dramatic way to categorize communication roadblocks of criticism, contempt, defensiveness, and stonewalling, which can chip away at connection. Here's a breakdown:

- **Criticism.** Attacking your partner's character, for example: "You never follow through on what you say you will do. I am the only one who can be relied on around here." This often includes the words *always* or *never*, and can result in your partner feeling assaulted, rejected, or hurt.

- **Contempt.** Examples include name-calling, mocking, hostile humor, and generally treating your partner with disrespect. This can be verbal (as in, "How hard is it to cook a meal? A child could do this better than you") or nonverbal (such as eye-rolling or scoffing). This behavior is the number-one predictor of divorce according to Gottman's research.
- **Defensiveness.** Typically a counterattack to perceived criticism; for example, "You're the one who made us late! You took too long getting ready." This often involves blaming your partner rather than taking responsibility for your contribution to a problem.
- **Stonewalling.** Shutting down and ignoring your partner when your body and brain get overwhelmed or "flooded"; refusing to engage in discussion; or even physically leaving a conflict.[16]

Add a screaming infant, juggling work and home, little-to-no sleep, and who knows what else, and a couple whose connection is shaky can be sent over the edge. Add that to your list of fears, right?

Dads: You Are Important!

One thing we learned in class that I did not expect, and that was really helpful down the road, was the important role fathers play. This is mostly going to apply to cisgender couples in different-sex relationships, so if you don't relate to that feel free to skip ahead. In essence, the research shows that most fathers want to be involved with their children, and that children whose fathers are intimately involved in their lives reap tons of benefits, including higher cognitive functioning, less risk of depression, better problem-solving skills, and higher overall life satisfaction.[17] Sounds pretty good, right? So why isn't every couple doing this? Turns out, there are actually several barriers that can prevent dads from being as involved as they want to be.

BARRIERS FOR DADS

- Dads may have shouldered the societal burden of being the family "provider" and may feel a strong need to focus on work to provide for their child, rather than being present with them.
- If the couple's relationship is strained, dads may withdraw from both their partner and their child.
- Gatekeeping behaviors from mom or partner that involve controlling who has access to the child and what they do with them can be a deterrent for dads.
- Feeling isolated or "on the outside looking in" if mom is the primary caregiver; lack of connection with other dads who may understand what they are going through.

WOMEN AS GATEKEEPERS

The biggest barriers that really made me think, and ultimately changed the way I approached things after our daughter was born, were the concepts of mothers acting as gatekeepers and the culture of women in general.[18] Let's break that down. Apparently, mothers, especially new mothers, can lean toward taking over a lot of control around who can have access to their child and what they do with them.

There are several reasons this might happen. It could be anxiety that something might go wrong with their baby; it might be a control thing in a situation where so much is out of control; or it could be that they don't trust their partner to do things the "right" way. I have seen friends who are worried that dad won't do things the "right" way or that something won't get taken care of, and the result is they do everything and dad ends up "helping," or helping as much as mom will let him. Try comparing that to a work situation. What if you had a coworker with whom you were collaborating on a project, and every time you did something, they hovered over you and told you to do it differently? What if they swooped in and took over every time it looked like you weren't 100 percent confident in a task? What would you do? Most of us would likely just hand over the reins. It's easier to give up than to continuously fight to be included.

Learning about this was an "aha" moment for me. Remember when we talked about fears and my worry about not being able to give up control? Here it was, right in front of me. This research was basically telling me that if I could not give up that control and let John build his own skills and relationship with our child, then I was preventing them from having a better connection and depriving my child of all of the proven benefits of that relationship. This was a *huge* motivator for me. Every time I saw something that felt not quite right and wanted to say something, every time I worried something wouldn't get done, I remembered that we were playing the long game, and a lot of the time I was able to at least keep my mouth shut, or refrain from jumping in and taking over.

There are also cultural factors that create barriers for dads. In the class, we learned that after babies are born, it is often the women in the community who come to give support and help mom. These can be friends, family members, neigh-bors, or coworkers. This gaggle of women, while so helpful in those new days, can also affect dad's relationship with the baby. Imagine if instead of just one gatekeeping mama, you were going up against two or three of them, all of whom had something to say every time you fumbled a diaper change, or who swooped in to do it themselves because you weren't doing it "right" or were struggling. What would you do? Give up? I would. I had never considered this social factor before, but it was absolutely true in my experience. When our daughter was born, who came to help? Our moms, and my sister-in-law. Male family members visited, but they weren't there to offer the support that the women gave. Knowing this ahead of time really helped me set expectations with those people who came to help us after our daughter was born. As a result, they gave both John and me space to mess up or struggle, but also offered advice or help when we asked. Because of this, we both got the opportunity to find our sea legs as parents: to put a diaper on wrong and suffer the con-sequences; to learn to comfort our daughter when she cried. Setting this tone in the early days helped establish a prece-dent that was really important to me—that just because I was mom did not make me the default parent when it came to baby care. I really didn't want to be the kind of couple where dad "babysat" or only did fun, playful things with the baby while mom did all of the caregiving tasks. I knew it would make me resentful, and that is a slippery slope for me as a partner and a parent.

John is just as capable of caring for our child as I am. Will he do it the same way? No. Is his way better or worse? No, just different. Is our child safe and loved and well taken care of? Absolutely. With this in mind, I was intentional about doing two things to help my husband build his own relationship and baby caretaking skills. The first was keeping my mouth shut. This is actually good to start practicing now, because as a parent you will have to learn when it is right to say something to your child and when it isn't. And it is really hard! The second was to give John and our daughter one-on-one time from very early on. Even if it was just leaving the house for an hour at first or going to take a shower. Those times when things just happen, and we have to figure them out, are what build confidence and skills. Most moms I know tend to get a lot of this time, but dads, not as much. Now that we have a three-year-old, John spends two days of the week with her while I work. It has been amazing to see their relationship grow and to watch them make their own rituals together. That would never have happened if they had not had that time together, just the two of them.

Other Strategies for Staying Connected

Attending class together got John and me talking about how we thought our relationship might change once we had a child. We discussed how we were going to have less time for ourselves and how we would have to be more intentional about connection. Before we had a kid, we would hang out a lot just the two of us, and could casually talk about things like scheduling, tasks, and big issues as they came up. This changed significantly after we had a baby, since we were juggling a lot more tasks and were just more stressed in general. We were busier overall, which left less time for the two of us together, and definitely less time for each of us to spend alone (goodbye solo *Gilmore Girls* marathons). As a couple, we had a few established pre-baby rituals that we leaned on a lot once we had a child.

- Family meeting once a week: a designated time to connect, discuss issues, and prepare for the week, during which we would:
  - Say one thing we appreciated about the other during the past week.
  - Talk about what we did well as a team, such as handling the change in routine when our family visited or communicating and staying consistent with boundaries that are important to us.
  - Review schedules and goals for the coming week: What is on the calendar and what do we need to get done?
  - Touch base on financial items and/or chores that need to be done.
  - Make a date-night plan: Who is planning this, what do we want to do?
  - Share what made each of us feel loved this past week; for example, "I felt loved when you made coffee for me before you went to work so that it was ready when I got up with the kids."
  - Ask each other "What stressors are coming up this week and how can I support you?" Answer might be: "I'm finishing a big project and might need to work late. Can you do bedtime on Tuesday and Wednesday while I work?"
  - Discuss any unresolved problems or challenges. This might be revisiting an argument from earlier in the week that is unresolved or bringing up a new topic.
  - End with a closing ritual like a kiss or saying I love you.
- Shared digital calendars and e-grocery/to-do lists, etc. really decrease conflicts about scheduling and food

shopping. We use Google Calendar and Google Keep for this.

- Prioritizing times to connect just the two of us, including:
  - Monthly date night
  - Scheduling sex

One thing that really keeps conflicts to a minimum is our weekly family meeting, a practice we picked up from a marriage conference we attended during our engagement and that has served us well over the years. It gives us a designated time to communicate with each other, review our schedules for the week, talk about things we need to get done, and air out any issues that remain unresolved. Another thing we do to stay connected is a monthly date night, which is built into our schedule with our nanny. Lastly, since becoming parents, we have scheduled sex. The window of opportunity for sex has narrowed considerably, and by the time we get to the end of the day we are often exhausted. Communicating this need and finding a time that works for both of us has helped us to continue having regular sex, which is really important for maintaining a sense of connection in our marriage. Initially we had a specific day of the week that we called "fun day" (as in Sunday fun day) that was our day to have sex. We typically would schedule sex during nap time in the afternoon, since the evening found us so drained. Now, with two kids and shifted schedules, that system doesn't work as well, so we will either check in with each other, saying something like "fun day tomorrow?" or will discuss it at our family meeting and work it into the schedule for the week. If we end up having sex in the evening it has to happen right after the kids go to bed. If I hit that couch in my pajamas with some dessert I am not getting back up for any sort of physical activity. It may sound boring, but the reality is that sponta-neous sex was a challenge even before we had kids, and it's now highly unlikely. If we want to continue to maintain inti-macy in this way, we need to schedule it. It takes intention and sometimes some creativity, but all of these things have been so helpful in nurturing our relationship through the transition of becoming parents.

Love Languages

I strongly urge you to think about the ways you and your spouse stay connected now and how those methods may continue or need to evolve after you have a baby. If you've never explored your own and your partner's love languages, that might be an exercise to do together to help maintain connection. Crash course: the "love languages" concept was created by Gary Chapman and outlines—very generally—the five different ways that people give and receive love. The five "languages" are:

- Words of Affirmation ("I love you.")
- Acts of Service ("I got the oil changed in your car, so you don't have to.")
- Giving or Receiving Gifts ("I picked up your favorite snack at the grocery store.")
- Quality Time ("Let's go on a walk together just the two of us.")
- Physical Touch ("Would you like a neck massage?")

The basic premise is that unless someone speaks your love language, the things they do to show love may not make you *feel* loved. If your language is Quality Time and your part-ner compliments you every day but never spends time with you, your tank isn't getting filled, for example. What language do you think you might show love through? What language do you think your partner might show love through? Are the ways you show love and like to receive love different?

In addition to exploring the specific ways you each give and receive connection, you can also explore the logistics of when you have time to connect. Do you make intentional time for each other, or does it just happen? Are you on opposite schedules, or do they line up pretty well? How much time do you spend together and how might that change (remember the pie chart)? Having a plan for staying connected after the baby arrives will decrease your stress by keeping your relationship with your partner strong. It is also helpful to look at how you and your partner currently make decisions and how you handle conflict. If you avoid conflict now, imagine how much more you will avoid it after a baby (babies make great excuses to avoid pretty much anything you want, by the way). If you and your partner struggle with making decisions together, think about all of the decisions you will have to make as parents and how difficult that might be. Take stock of your relationship and see if there are any things that need adjusting. You want to be as strong as you can be going into parenthood, because it tests your relationship like nothing else.

We've covered some pretty serious topics so far, so let's shift to something positive. Think about the characteristics in your partner that will make them a great parent. When I thought about John, I called to mind how patient and even-tempered he is, and how he is great at being silly and playing. These are all fantastic qualities in toddlerland, and I am sure they will continue to come in handy as the years go on. Acknowledging your partner's strengths allows you to give them more grace and helps you maintain perspective when they struggle in areas that don't come as naturally.

Ideas from Other Parents

I asked parents how they continued to nurture their relationship after they had a child. They had some great ideas, which I'll share here:

- "We give each other time alone to recharge."
- "We go to counseling to remember how to communicate and prioritize each other."
- "We communicate, talk through our feelings, and support each other."
- "We find time to spend just the two of us in the evenings after the kids are asleep."
- "We schedule time to talk, and plan days ahead to have sex."
- "We do date nights, and a few times a year we get an overnight sitter and go to a hotel to reconnect, sleep in, etc."
- "We take trips together just the two of us."
- "We go on day dates while the kids are in school."
- "We try to talk in the evenings rather than just zoning out in front of the TV."
- "We ask each other one question each night before bed from a list of questions we found online, which helps us learn new things about each other."

Next Steps

This might seem like a lot to add to your to-do list of ways to ensure you are a good parent. The good news is that just being aware of these patterns is the starting line to improving the strength of your connection. To explore more, take a look at the recommended books and courses in the Resources section at the back of the book, and consider seeking the help of a counselor. As we have already established, parenting is a huge transition laden with stress, sleep deprivation, and hopes and fears. It can't hurt to have a professional on your team just in case you need it. When John and I moved, we went to some sessions with a counselor to talk through the transition, and I now feel reassured knowing we can call her if we need her again.

Summary

- The transition to parenthood inevitably changes your relationship with your partner. These changes may be beneficial, involving an increased bond and communication, or challenging, as there is less time together and more potential for conflict.

- It's important to maintain connection in your relationship. Research shows that the stress of parenting can further erode relationships already undergoing challenges.

- According to research, dad's involvement leads to many long-term benefits for their children, but barriers like pressure to provide and maternal gatekeeping can prevent them from being as involved as they may like.

- The marriage experts Drs. John and Julie Gottman recommend two things to help couples maintain satisfaction during the transition of having children:

continues ›

1. Both partners should be involved in pregnancy and birth, and with the new baby.
2. Couples must make an effort to maintain connection and prioritize their relationship.

- Take stock of the ways you and your partner stay connected now and think about how those may need to be adjusted after your baby arrives.

- Consider seeing a counselor as a couple early on to establish a potential resource for the transition to parenting.

Discussion Topics:
Transition

1. How do you think having a child will change your relationship?

2. How do you think your day-to-day life will change?

3. How will you stay connected after you have a child?

4. How do you currently handle conflict?

5. How do you make decisions together?

6. Would it be helpful for you to see a counselor together to discuss issues, learn better communication skills, or establish a relationship for support after your baby arrives?

7. Make a list of qualities that will make your partner a great parent. Share the list with them.

Attachment: When History Repeats Itself

"What a child doesn't receive
he can seldom later give."

—P.D. JAMES

ATTACHMENT HISTORY. WE all have it. It dictates how we interact in relationships with other human beings pretty much every minute of every day. Attachment theory originated in the 1960s with Dr. John Bowlby, a British psychiatrist, and has since developed into the scientific basis for how we understand human relationships. Attachment is formed primarily in our first few years of life. It works like this: Our experiences with our primary caregivers (often our parents) during the first few years of life hardwire in our brain how we relate to people, and unless we intentionally do something to change this framework, we use it in relationships for the rest of our lives. Left unaware of our attachment history, we can't truly understand the nature of how we connect with others.

We all have emotional baggage we carry around in life that can be tied to our relationships with our parents. Some of it might be helpful to our lives, such as developing a strong work ethic, organizational skills, or the ability to make small talk with others. Some of it might be hindering or challenging; for example, an intolerance of imperfections or differences, an insecurity that makes us doubt our relationships, or a constant need for control. Our first connections with our earliest caregivers build a framework that we carry with us through childhood and into adulthood and that becomes the lens through which we see the world; this in turn affects our behaviors. These connections also contribute to the framework of our parenting, whether we are aware of it or not. As parents, we do what we know, and what we know is our own history and our interactions with our parents when we were children. The goal of this chapter is to introduce you to the concept of attachment, help you explore what your attachment style might be, and understand how that will likely affect your parenting. Note: For simplicity's sake, I will be using the word *parents* to refer to the primary caregivers in a child's life. I recognize that many people didn't grow up with two parents or were possibly raised by other family members or adults who weren't their parents.

Let's take my childhood as a case study in how attachment can develop. I was raised by a single mom and grew up in a household that valued strength and independence. I am a self-reliant, confident, and assertive woman. I consider this to be advantageous most of the time—except, you know, when it isn't. Even though my mom was loving, caring, and involved in my life, I picked up some spoken and unspoken messages along the way. Somewhere, for example, I internalized the message "If you have a problem, you better handle it yourself." By the time I was a teenager, if I messed up, my first instinct was to hide it and try to fix it myself. Like the time my car got towed at school because I used the high school parking lot without a parking pass. Did I call my mom and ask for help? Nope. I had a friend drive me home to pick up a huge jar of change I had collected, then took it to the bank to cash it in for bills, and then headed to the impound to bail my car out. I never told my mom until I was at least in college, if not older. Would she have been upset if I told her about it when it happened? Probably. Would she have helped me? Absolutely. Likely the worst that would have happened is I would have had to do chores to work off the payment or received a stern lecture. It definitely wasn't rational, but my internal voice told me this was something I needed to avoid and take care of on my own.

I carry some of these habits into adulthood. If I am having a hard time with something, often I will work through it on my own until I feel comfortable enough to share it with John. The vulnerability of asking for help before I feel like I have a handle on things still feels unsafe to me somehow. As a person in a relationship, and as a parent, this is something that is important for me to be aware of. I want my child to know they can come to me when they are in trouble or have a problem. I don't want them to be like me and think they have to handle everything on their own.

Types of Attachment

Let's talk about different kinds of attachment and what they mean. Keep in mind a few things as you explore this section. One, attachment is a spectrum: You may see yourself in one category or another, but we all have the ability to flow between categories and experience differing levels of intensity. Two, attachment is changeable. This chapter might bring up all sorts of worries or difficult feelings for you, but that doesn't mean you can't work through them. The first step is awareness, which I hope you gain here. And lastly, remember that **there does not exist anywhere in the world a parent who is perfect**. That means that you won't be a perfect parent no matter how hard you try, and it means that no matter how wonderful your parents were, they weren't perfect either. We all have challenging aspects to our histories. Now, let's dive in.

Early research described attachment as a set of static categories; you either fit into one or the other. But as research has evolved, so has the science of attachment. Attachment is now described as a spectrum. Imagine a color spectrum with green in the middle, blue to the left, and red to the right. That green middle ground is the ideal world of secure attachment, where things are balanced, integrated, and generally working well. Shift to the left and we've entered the cool blue zone of dismissive attachment. Cool as a cucumber, dismissive attachment often means concealing or shutting down emotions and being ever in control. As children, we learned that our needs would be overlooked, so we took them into our own hands, which usually meant suppressing them. Moving all the way over to the right, we visit the heated territory of entangled attachment. Intensity and desperation for connection lead to hyper-emotional interactions. We learned that our caregivers might be there for us sometimes, but other times might not. This resulted in us cleaving to them for dear life whenever we had the opportunity to connect, for fear that they would leave us again. These three are considered "organized" types of attachment; there is also disorganized attachment, which occurs when an attachment figure is unsafe and the brain can't process the primal need for safety and connection at the same time, which often results in erratic behavior.

To make these categories more accessible, and also because a lot of millennials I know are Disneyphiles, I'll give a Disney movie correlation to each attachment type.

- **Secure attachment** is the holy grail of attachment. It is what we all strive toward if we lean toward another category. Secure attachment occurs when your parents were able to clearly see, interpret, and meet your needs consistently when you were a child. You learned that your parents were safe and there for you if you needed them. If this was your family growing up, emotions were likely encouraged and were viewed in a positive light.

  Disney movie: *Moana.* First of all, girl has two parents who don't die—rare in a Disney flick. Second, her parents guide and support her. Even when they don't understand Moana's desires or behaviors, they care for her and eventually come together in support of her mission to explore and grow in her own identity. Her grandmother also plays a big part in this—a great example of how attachment figures aren't always parents.

- **Dismissive attachment** applies to us strong and independent types. Dismissive attachment occurs when your parents misinterpret, brush off, or don't meet your needs consistently as a child. You internalize self-reliance, independence, and often control. You can't always depend on others to meet your needs, so you decide to only depend on yourself. Emotions, especially messy negative ones like sadness, shame, and fear, are dangerous, because they can make you feel vulnerable and weak. Those with dismissive attachment styles tend to "dismiss" or avoid these emotions.

When they are distressed, they will usually turn toward an outward experience like exercise, working overtime, or food or alcohol to help them rather than relying on another person.

Disney movie: *Frozen.* Kid has ice powers. Kid's parents don't understand her ice powers and her powers are scary at times, so their solution is to just shut it down. Trade "ice powers" for "messy emotions" and you've got classic dismissive attachment. Elsa's journey is actually a fantastic metaphor for what happens when we suppress emotions. We can work hard to hide them and stuff them away, but eventually they are going to explode all over people, often at an inopportune time. If we learn to embrace them and feel them, we can learn healthy ways of expression and processing that allow us to move with our emotions instead of against them.

- **Entangled attachment** applies to those whose emotions seem to run high. All. The. Time. The scientific literature uses the terms "entangled" and "preoccupied" interchangeably for this category, which can be confusing. I prefer "entangled" because I picture a child and parent all tangled up in each other's emotions, unable to escape. Entangled attachment occurs when as a child your parents see and meet your needs sometimes, and other times don't, and you don't know what you will get at any given moment. You learn that when you have a person's attention or affection you have to desperately attempt to keep it, otherwise it will disappear on you. You become hyper-focused on or preoccupied with maintaining that connection. Emotions—especially the loud and messy ones—can become tools to manipulate those close to you into staying with you. You may struggle to maintain independence in close relationships and may have difficulty making decisions for fear of damaging your relationship.

Disney movie: *Tangled.* Child's "adoptive mother" (which pains me to write), locks her in a tower, using child's magic hair to meet her need of being forever youthful. This is some twisted *Hocus Pocus* shit, but Mother Gothel is a clear example of the entangled parent. She literally won't let her child leave her and goes to great lengths to make the outside world seem like an unsafe place so that her child will want to stick close by. Rapunzel struggles throughout the movie to recognize her own needs while meeting the needs of her mother. *The movie is even called* Tangled. Too perfect.

· **Disorganized attachment** is often found in those who had a traumatic experience as a child, like abuse or neglect, or even something like the death of a parent. Disorganized attachment occurs when your parents are a source of fear or are absent or unsafe. You learn that your safe place can turn frightening at any moment. Your brain cannot process this paradox, and so it struggles. You may be triggered by past trauma or develop mental health concerns. Those with disorganized attachment styles may struggle to connect with others, and when they are distressed their behavior may look erratic or "disorganized."

Disney movie: *The Little Mermaid.* Teenager with a dead mom and overbearing dad gives up her family and basically her entire identity to pursue a romantic relationship with a dude she met once while he was unconscious—you know, every parent's dream for their child. The sure signifier of disorganized attachment is the struggle in forming and maintaining relationships. This often involves trying to attach to anyone you come into contact with, desperately seeking safety even with a stranger. Ariel is a good example of this. Yeah, you could write it off as teenage rebellion, or you could think about how signing over your entire life after getting into one yelling match with your dad in an attempt to seduce a prince means there's probably something deeper going on there. Also, she gets married at the end of the story. She's *sixteen*! I need to stop thinking about this because it's ruining childhood for me.

ATTACHMENT EXERCISE

Review the questions below and think through or jot down what comes to mind. Don't analyze it too much; think more stream of consciousness—whatever comes to mind when you read the question. It can be general or specific. This is just to give you some idea of where you may fall on the attachment spectrum.

1. What is your first memory of your mother/father/primary caregiver?
2. List five adjectives that describe your relationship with your mother/father/primary caregiver.
3. During your childhood, what happened if you were sick? Injured? Hurt?
4. How did your parents or primary caregivers express love, anger, disappointment?
5. As an adult, do you tend to seek people out when you are stressed or avoid them?

I want to be clear that this exercise does not constitute a diagnosis, and that you won't necessarily know definitively what your true attachment style is just by answering these questions. Attachment is complex. The only true way to know where you fall on the attachment spectrum is to undergo a full adult attachment history assessment with a trained clinician. However, you can get *a sense* of your attachment style by exploring and reflecting on your own history and interactions in current and past relationships.

All of that being said, let's break down what your answers may look like and where you might be on the spectrum.

You might fall toward the "secure" part of the spectrum if:

- You were able to list both positive and negative things about your childhood.
- When you were young, your parents were present and comforting when you were sick or hurt.
- Your parents expressed love, anger, and disappointment in appropriate ways without making you responsible for those emotions.
- You grew up in a home where most of the time expectations and consequences were clear and life was predictable overall.

You might fall toward the "dismissive" part of the spectrum if:

- You only listed positive things about your childhood and parents, or had a hard time remembering things at all.
- You remember being told to "walk it off" or "suck it up" or "you're fine" when you were sick, injured, or hurt as a child.

- Your parents easily expressed positive emotions like love or pride but disconnected when it came to more complicated emotions like disappointment or sadness.
- Your parents highly encouraged independence and self-sufficiency; being needy was seen as a weakness or flaw.

You might fall toward the "entangled" part of the spectrum if:

- You have many intense memories of your mother or father from early childhood.
- Your parents made you responsible for their emotions, and you had to walk on eggshells to make sure you didn't upset them.
- Family interactions tended to get heated quickly.
- Your parents were extra attentive when you were sick or hurt.
- Your parents struggled when you tried to disconnect from them or explore more independence, perhaps becoming manipulative to keep you close.

You might have "disorganized" attachment features if:

- Your childhood relationships with your parents included connection but also significant safety risks like abuse or neglect.
- You find yourself triggered in relationships and unable to fully connect.
- You have competing instincts to both seek connection with your loved ones and turn away from them and only rely on yourself.

Anyone worried yet? Thinking about how much your parents messed you up? Making an appointment with your therapist? Great. So, what happens if your attachment style is not ideal? Are you doomed to be a bad parent? Not at all.

The good news is that there is a secret fifth kind of attachment called "earned secure attachment." Even if you experienced insecure attachment in childhood, as an adult you can do the work to process your childhood experience to make sense of your attachment story and how it affects your current relationships.[19] This is often called "inner-child" work and can be done in a variety of ways, including doing reflective work, talking with a therapist, and talking with a partner or close friend. One tricky aspect to this concept is that often we don't know that we have attachment stuff that is being triggered until we are actually parents, and our kid does something that pushes that button. In the mental health world, a "trigger" refers to something that causes you distress or to feel overwhelmed. It is often linked to an experience you may have had as a child. For example, if as a child your parents were strict about being tidy, then mess may be triggering to you now. In the parenting world, I think a trigger is often something that brings up significant fear for you or causes you to lose your cool with your kid. This can be small and subtle, so the first step to discovering a trigger is to pay attention to how you react in challenging situations with your child. You'll start to notice patterns, and then you can reflect on those to see if you can determine the cause of the trigger. If you flip every time your kid yells at you, it might be flashing you back to when you were yelled at as a child. If you are hyper-focused on what your child eats and find yourself getting into power struggles over it, you might explore your own relationship with food and how your parents handled that with you.

If you clearly know you have some attachment history that you need to take a look at now, dive into that before you have a kid. If you aren't sure, just have it on your radar. When you encounter something with your child that is really bothering you, ask yourself if it might be connected to something from your own childhood. Often it is. We tend to be triggered the most when our kids exhibit behaviors that were unacceptable for us to have as children. Sorting this out is easier said than done, and might even be painful, depending on what your relationship was like with your parents. We'll explore this more in chapter 8, when we tackle discipline and parenting styles; for now, know that the payoff of exploring our own attachment struggles allows us to be fully present with our children, bringing us peace and greater closeness.

Becoming a parent will send you on your own attachment journey whether you want to go or not. It's not just you and your kid, it's you and your parents—and their parents as well. Being aware of your history and how it affects your parenting is key. If you take one thing away from this book, let it be this: To be the best versions of ourselves as parents, we need to do our own work to understand how our attachment history can affect our child. The number-one cause of struggle I see in the parents I work with is when their child has triggered something from their own attachment history. Sometimes parents are aware of it and can do the work to explore their struggle and heal that part of their inner child. Sometimes they continue to be in denial and end up blaming their child's behaviors for their reaction, slowly pushing away their child and losing compassion for them in the process.

My personal goal is to make sure I mess up my kids in a completely different way than my parents messed me up, so at least we are doing something new! In all seriousness though, I feel an important part of parenting is learning from the mistakes and missteps of those who came before us. And if you can't acknowledge what those were, you're letting your history drive the bus.

Childhood Hurts = Adult Struggles

One experience from my own childhood perfectly illustrates the concept of how attachment stays with us and affects our behavior as adults. Some of you may have experienced something similar. From when I was about three to when I was about nine, my mom and I lived with her partner at the time, who we will call Kate. I have no idea how much experience Kate had with children before becoming a stepparent, but regardless, she was in that role to some extent in our family. Kate was a police officer and worked off-hours, so I was sometimes at home with her during the day while my mom was at work. When my mom was home, she was always the primary parent, so things were fine. Expectations were high, but reasonable and clear. Rules and consequences were logical and made sense. I don't recall her raising her voice (she was more of a say-it-through-clenched-teeth kind of parent).

But when I was alone with Kate, things weren't fine. Kate had high and unreasonable expectations for a child my age. She expected me to be seen and not heard. She got angry if I was too demanding or if I bothered her. If I made a mistake or broke a rule, as school-aged children tend to do, she would demand to know *why* I did it. I would mumble "I don't know," which would really set her off. I can still hear the words "'I don't know' is *not* an acceptable answer!" in the exact angry tone in which she threw them at me. On days when I was home alone with her, I took to staying in my sunshine-yellow bedroom, sleeping until at least noon to avoid interactions during which I would inevitably do something to set her off. My most traumatizing memory of this time comes from when I was about eight, and I was out with her at the mall running errands. I had to use the bathroom but didn't want to bother her, so I just kept holding it. I think you can guess how that ended up. Yep. I wet myself in a department store. On top of the shame of wetting myself in public, I was berated for the inconvenience and told that I had better be careful not to ruin the upholstery in Kate's truck. I had to ride home sitting on a trash bag in my wet clothes, filled to the brim with shame.

This story is still painful for me to tell, and to this day my mom and I haven't really talked about that time in detail (there's some dismissive attachment for you). My guess is that she figured out what was happening, and likely was experiencing similar interactions with Kate herself. However it happened, Kate and my mom separated when I was nine or ten, and I never spoke with Kate again. It wasn't until I was an adult that I recognized those interactions for the emotional abuse they were.

It's been more than twenty years, but I still carry the effects of that time with me. Making a mistake puts me instantly into a shame spiral, which is why I spend so much time and energy planning, researching, and trying to predict outcomes. The refrain of "'I don't know' is not an acceptable answer" pushes me to search for reasons for everything, from behavior to relationship struggles to the nonsensical happenings in the world. To this day, when I am on a home visit or out with other people, I debate whether to inconvenience them with a request to use the bathroom. Order, routine, and predictability are my comfort, because without them I am not safe. Or so my eight-year-old self says.

Yes, I had this difficult and painful experience as a child, and yes it affects me still. But here's the thing: I don't want my history driving the bus when it comes to my parenting decisions, so I've done the work. I've talked with therapists; I've explored my own feelings. I've been through the adult attachment interview as part of my training and received my spectrum spot of secure/dismissive. I've identified the parts of my history that may get triggered for me as a parent so that I can be aware and choose how I react. Doing the work helped me make sense of those childhood experiences so that I don't carry them with me day to day. I don't feel that same rush of shame when my own child makes a mistake. I don't have unrealistic expectations for her. I recognize when I'm frustrated if she makes a mess I have to clean up or has a meltdown that makes me feel out of control, and I work through that feeling so it doesn't drive my decisions and behavior. I know my story may sound a bit extreme, and you might be thinking, *I didn't experience abuse as a child, so I am probably fine.* (Side note: "Fine" is a dismissive person's favorite feeling, and, spoiler . . . it's not a feeling). Let's look at an experience from my husband's life that might seem more typical.

John and I both fall into the range of secure/dismissive attachment. We share a lot of characteristics in this area. We were raised primarily by single mothers, and both of us value independence. Both of us struggle with showing emotions and have initial instincts to keep them inside. Both of us are hesitant to be vulnerable. When we talked about our histories together and what we felt led to this hesitancy in each of us, he told me a story that stuck with me. When he was younger, he and his brothers had a lot of conflict (siblings, am I right?). As the middle child, he was between an older brother who liked to instigate and a younger one who was full of anger and easy to set off. John talked about how his older brother would get his younger one all riled up and then basically let him loose, with John as the target for agitation, anger, or fights. As a result, he developed behaviors to cope. One of these is that he trained himself not to be ticklish. Seriously. It's not that he doesn't feel it. He just holds it in. You can tickle him forever, and he will just sit there. No wiggles, no laughs. With a devoted and caring but overwhelmed mother, these three boys were not uncommonly left to fend for themselves when experiencing conflict. John's ability to not react to a tickle, poke, or insult was his way of surviving, and it worked well for him. He needed it to get through those years. In case you are wondering, he and his brothers are all grown up now and very close. As far as I know, they don't have physical altercations anymore! As an only child, this whole situation baffles me, but I clearly know very little about how sibling dynamics work—as my husband has informed me many times.

How does this translate to functioning in adulthood? John still hides his emotions, and things just don't seem to affect him. That's part of what makes him a great air traffic controller, so it is a strength in some ways. In other ways, it is a struggle. In our marriage, I feel like I am often prying his emotions out of him. If he is angry, he tends to clam up until he has worked through it on his own, and only then will he talk about it. If he is sad, he holds it in. I have only seen him cry twice. One of the most beautiful memories I have is him insisting on not seeing me on our wedding day until I walked down the aisle in my dress. I remember him tearing up, and there is a photo from our wedding of his face, full of emotion, as he gazes at me coming toward him. In hindsight, I see what a beautiful offering this was to me, that this man chose to bestow the gift of vulnerability and being emotionally demonstrative upon me in that moment. It is rare, and I get to keep it forever.

John and I have the benefit of having similar experiences to draw from. I also struggle with showing emotions, so I understand the need to keep it together, to not seem needy or weak. We work on it with each other. We've had to be intentional in getting comfortable with our daughter's big emotions and working through those with her rather than trying to shut them down with a "you're fine," distracting her from them, or ignoring them.

What Other Parents Said

I asked the parents I interviewed what has come up for them from their history with their parents since they had a kid—and boy did they deliver.

RECOGNIZING TRIGGERS

"I had a yeller for a mother. I found myself falling into that pattern as my kids left toddlerhood and started growing up. I have fought very, very hard to overcome that. I think about my relationship with my mom a lot. I believe she loved me as I love my kids, but our relationship is difficult now. I contemplate the reasons she may have made the decisions she did."

"My mom always did everything for us, and I catch myself trying to do everything for my daughter instead of letting her struggle sometimes and figure it out. I am also very task-oriented, and it is hard for me to give her space to figure things out. My dad would raise his voice when he was upset, and I still have a reaction to that as an adult when my husband raises his voice at our child, which makes me go into protective mode."

EMOTIONAL BURDENS

"My mother was a young mom and was an extremely avoidant mom. She didn't do emotion, she didn't teach us what that was, and we were really encouraged to be independent, meet our own needs, and be self-sufficient. That has come up for me more in the toddler years. The meltdowns really trigger dismissiveness for me, to where if I am not in a good place I will walk away, which will escalate my daughter's tantrums. I notice that when I am not in a healthy place my mom will come out in me and I will just shut down."

CONNECTIONS

"My mom is a real nurturer, and now, being a mom, I want to be that way as well. Because I had that kind of a mom it is easier for me to do that."

"One thing my mom always did a good job of was having a relationship with me where I could come to her with anything and there was no judgment. Even though my kids are little still, I try to not let my face show if I am disappointed and just sit down and hear what they have to say."

"My parents always did a really good job of making mundane day-to-day things fun through singing songs or doing something silly, and that is something I try to do with my son. Have fun even if we are just doing mundane things like cleaning up or going to school."

PARENT PRESENCE

"I was raised with a traditional dad who went to work and a mom who mostly stayed home, and I wanted to be more

emotionally present than my dad was and be more involved than he was. My dad also traveled a lot and I wanted to be sure our kids had both of their parents present."

"My mom worked a lot when I was a child and was a single mom by the time I was five, so I try to be really intentional about being present and connecting with my son."

"I remember being so irritated as a kid whenever my mom or dad would be tired and not want to take me places, and now I get where they were coming from, but I want to do better than that. I might be tired, but this is her one childhood, so I suck it up and do the things they want to do."

"My dad was kind of cold when I was growing up. He said 'I love you' and hugged me, but always seemed to keep an emotional barrier between us. I don't know if it was something with his expectation about what masculinity should be, or if he had some sort of wounds from his own childhood. This has had a huge impact on how I parent."

HIGH EXPECTATIONS

"I had a single mom, and everything that she did, I more or less do the opposite. She was not a great mom across the board. I catch myself sounding like her—like she was OCD about cleaning, bed making, etc.—and I have to stop myself and realize I am being too hard on my children. I apologize to them when I mess up and talk about how I want to do better. My mom was supportive of things only if she liked what I was doing, and I focus on supporting my kids whether I am interested in the thing or not."

"I tend to consistently use my own experiences of being a child in order to understand what my three-year-old is feeling in any given situation. I'm a big feeler with lots of emotions and

I think a lot of my emotions growing up have somehow stuck in my sense memory. I can remember how frustrating it is to be a kid and have some adults who are constantly expecting you to not act like a kid when it suits them. I still fall into this trap sometimes and find myself having unrealistic expectations that I have to give myself a reality check for."

"Growing up we had high expectations, like doing well in school, and I think that I incorporate that in my parenting. I've merged my stricter upbringing with the more liberal way my husband was parented. I realized my strict upbringing was a little too much pressure."

CHILDHOOD TRAUMA

"My family was pretty dysfunctional, and my dad was an alcoholic. At seventeen I had to get a job and grow up really quickly. My mom was a 'Don't cry or I'll give you something to cry about' type of person. My emotions were not validated. I think parenting brings out all of your childhood trauma. I think about my kids and how I want them to never feel like they have to take care of me, and not be 'parentified' like I was. I really want them to enjoy being kids."

"I have had to go to lots of therapy because I was a victim of sexual trauma as a child, so I am hypersensitive to it. I've had to really work on that, not pathologizing things like her wetting herself and projecting things onto her. I am also way more adamant about body safety than I think I would be otherwise."

CULTURAL INFLUENCES

"My parents worked a lot, and in summer we couldn't afford daycare. So, my parents would drop us off at the library and we would stay there all day, and that is how I fell in love with books.

*I have invested in that with my son. My parents also encouraged
a strong faith, which I have passed on. I also want to celebrate
my culture, and I want my son to know that he is Nigerian, and I
focus on that more than my parents do."*

*"We have this interesting dynamic where our families are very
different. My Hispanic heritage comes with a lot of traditions,
or things that I find important or want to do, and my husband's
family had a lot less of that; they are much more go with the flow.
I have to think about if I am doing this because we have always
done it, or is it really something I want to do with my kid?"*

*"Culturally, Vietnamese families don't like to show feelings.
When I was a child I cried and was scolded. And now it is
different. When our kids cry, we find out why they are crying,
and comfort them."*

*"The differences in how we were both raised became more
apparent once we had kids. Visiting my husband's family in
Nigeria helped me understand more how he was raised and
navigate that as parents. My dad was pretty involved when I
was a child, so I had that expectation for my husband as a dad
as well. I think my willingness to be a stay-at-home mom was
influenced by my mom also doing that."*

Knowing Better and Doing Better

Notice the variety of answers here. Some people remembered great things about their parents that they wanted to
do with their own children. A lot had painful experiences or
simply things they felt were missing from their own childhood that they were determined to do differently or avoid.
One surprise for me was hearing parents talk about how their
own childhood experience influenced the way they expected
their partner to parent. Let's say your parents were divorced,

and your dad would sometimes show up for his weekends with you and sometimes bail. You might have very high expectations that your partner will follow through on his commitments with your child. It may even be triggering for you if your partner misses something they said they would be there for, even if it's not a regular habit. It could take you right back to that feeling of abandonment you experienced as a child with your dad. If you aren't aware of it, you might end up taking all of your anger, sadness, and other big feelings associated with that experience and projecting them onto your partner. Heavy stuff, right? If you have an experience from childhood that is going to affect how you feel your partner should be as a mom or dad, *please* talk to them about this. This is a burden they can share with you, but only if you invite them to do so. Imagine all of your issues being triggered by the way your partner interacts with your child, and them not even being aware of it. Recipe for disaster, right?

"Why should I care about all of this psychobabble?" you might ask. You should care because you are planning to become a parent, and your kids will inherit whatever attachment baggage you carry around unless you do the work to shed that baggage and parent from a different place. Or as Dr. Vanessa Lapointe says in her book *Parenting Right From the Start: Laying a Healthy Foundation in the Baby and Toddler Years:* "You cannot . . . give to your child what you did not get in your own childhood—unless you are willing to acknowledge those gaps and work to fill them in."[20] All of the research on attachment backs this up. For instance, a study done with foster parents in the United Kingdom showed that children placed in new foster homes took on the attachment of their primary caregiver in just *three months.*[21]

Here's the thing: If we don't do the work, if we choose to hide from our past, or bury it deep inside and ignore it, it will still get uncovered by this mystical experience we call parenting. One of the most remarkable and at the same time infuriating things about being a parent is that your children will unearth things for you that may have remained dormant for years. Sometimes this can be wonderful, like bringing out your silly side, or reigniting a passion you had as a child when your kid gets into the same thing. But it can also be agonizing, say, when your child brings out the yeller in you that you swore you would never be, or hits you in the midst of a meltdown and flashes you back to the abuse you experienced as a child. Either way, it's coming for you. Parenthood exposes all of your vulnerabilities whether you want it to or not. And you can either get on board and work through your stuff, or you can try to avoid it and let it take you over. I've seen this countless times in the parents I work with. There's the mom whose eleven-year-old daughter would yell hurtful things at her when she was angry, bringing up the anger she herself felt as a child and was punished for by her parents. The dad whose seven-year-old has a meltdown on the playground and his gut response is shame and embarrassment because as a child he was told it was not okay to cry. The majority of us have childhood pain that may very likely be triggered by our own children. So, what can you do to break the cycle?

- Explore your own attachment.
- Take the short quiz in this chapter. While unlikely to be definitive, it can give you a sense of where you fall on the spectrum of attachment.
- If you want to go deeper, find a practitioner to do a full adult attachment interview with you. I promise, it will be eye-opening.
- Read books on the subject, such as *The Power of Showing Up.*

- Talk with your spouse.
- Journal about your childhood experiences.
- Find a therapist to do some inner-child work with you.
- Explore the Enneagram, a personality test that is linked to childhood wounds. This has been helpful to me in growing my self-awareness and connecting my childhood experiences to my adult behaviors. There are nine personality types in the Enneagram and I am a 1, which is often called the "perfectionist" or the "reformer." I am constantly looking at how to improve things; I will go to great lengths to avoid a mistake, and I have a "right" way of doing things, even if it is just something I made up. Learning this about myself has helped me put words to some of my behaviors, dig deeper on what motivations are driving them, and catch myself when I am reacting from a place of stress. If you are interested in exploring the Enneagram for yourself, I recommend reading *The Road Back to You* by Ian Morgan Cron and Suzanne Stabile.

Why take a journey to explore your past and examine how it affects your present? As a parent, I want to learn to be comfortable in my child's emotions. I want my children to celebrate and see the function of all emotions—the good, the bad, and the ugly. This is different from how I was parented, and it is a lot of work. But it is oh so worth it. I believe we have the power to change generational dysfunction if we summon the courage to be vulnerable and look inside ourselves.

Summary

- Attachment history is baggage we carry around in life that is determined by our relationships with our parents or primary caregivers. Some of it is positive and some of it is negative. It affects how we connect with others in all of our relationships, especially with our children.

- The attachment styles are secure, dismissive, entangled, and disorganized. Although we may lean toward one style or category, the spectrum of attachment is fluid and changeable.

- Being aware of your attachment history and challenges is the first step to "earned security" that can prevent you from passing the same challenges on to your child.

- If you experienced emotional pain or trauma around attachment in your childhood, it is your responsibility to do the work to make sense of those experiences and how they may affect your parenting.

- You may have experiences from your childhood that also influence how you expect your partner to parent. It is important to share these in order to be on the same page, and for your partner to be aware of your potential attachment triggers or sensitivities.

- All of the challenges from your childhood are going to be brought up when you become a parent, whether you want them to or not. You can either explore and work through them, or you can let them drive your reactions and behaviors.

Discussion Topics:
Attachment

1. Where do you think you and your partner might fall on the attachment spectrum?

2. Where do you think your parents fell on the attachment spectrum? What about your partner's parents?

3. What do you think parenting will bring up for you from your childhood history?

4. Do you have any experiences from your childhood that might influence how you expect your partner to parent?

5. As a parent, what do you think you might do that is just like your mom or dad (or other primary caregiver)? This can be positive or negative.

6. What aspects of your own history might pose a challenge for you as a parent?

Roles: The Division of Labor after *Actual* Labor

"Individually, we are one drop.
Together, we are an ocean."

—RYUNOSUKE SATORO

WHEN IT CAME to planning for parenthood, I insisted on talking about the division of labor before our child arrived. I am a feminist and an independent person, and I didn't want to get lost in the shuffle of becoming the primary parent for our child just because I happened to have a vagina and got the label of "mom."

I am fortunate that my husband is also a feminist, although I'm not sure he would claim the description. We discussed roles and responsibilities early on and came to an agreement on expectations for the beginning of our parenting journey. It was important to both of us that we each be involved as much as possible and share the parenting load. We both went to all of my doctor's appointments when I was pregnant and discussed decisions together. John was right by my side through labor and birth, which turned out to be one of the most intimately bonding experiences of our marriage. In the days after our daughter was born, my jobs were to figure out breastfeeding and help my body heal, and John did pretty much everything else. We alternated getting up at night to soothe her back to sleep when she woke, even when I did all of the feedings because, boobs. We both wanted to be capable of caring for our child alone if needed and started that early on. One thing that really helped was that John had an odd schedule. His days off were during the week, so he had the baby on those days, and I had her on weekends. This gave us each one-on-one bonding time with her and opportunities to figure things out on our own.

Now, I am not going to pretend that things have just gone swimmingly in this area. I don't think John took our daughter anywhere outside our house by himself until she was over a year old, and we've had some tearful hormone- and patriarchy-induced conflicts about sharing the load. But generally, we've been on the same page about what we wanted our parenting roles to look like because we talked about it before we jumped into the deep end of feedings, diapers, and night wake-ups.

A note on breastfeeding: I was able to breastfeed my daughter for the first year of her life. It was what I wanted to do going in, and I am grateful that my body and her body were able to do that together. We are clear that I am *grateful*, yes? Okay. Even though there were many positives to it, for me, breastfeeding was a huge burden. It consumed my life and added a constant current of anxiety underneath that first year. I was always calculating when the baby would eat again, how much, if I needed to pump, and if it was worth pumping or if I could sleep/go out/take a break, etc. I also resented that this was the one thing John could not do. Sure, he could give the baby a bottle, and he did. But even doing that was often the same amount of work—or more—for me because I had to pump to have the milk for the bottle, and then pump again during the feeding to keep my body on the same production schedule. If I was there, it just made more sense to nurse. It really bothered me that just because I was a woman, I had this burden that John would never have. I wanted to share this because I expect there are others who feel the same way, and I want you to know that it's okay to choose breastfeeding and not be in love with it, or even happy about it sometimes. It is, of course, also okay to love it, or to not choose it at all. A fed baby is a healthy and happy baby, no matter how you go about it.

You Do You

Talking with other parents, I've come to find that everyone divides their roles and responsibilities differently, and that there are many factors that go into these decisions. Job flexibility, childcare options, gender roles and expectations, and general confidence in ability are just a few of them. Some heterosexual couples split along gender lines, with the female partner taking on a lot of the childcare and inside housework, and the male partner working more, doing yard work, and grilling (I can't tell you how many times I've had to keep a straight face when a dude tells me in an interview that he shares cooking responsibilities—a.k.a. stands outside over a grill five times a year to make one part of a meal and drink while his wife does everything else). Some couples outsource a lot of their household work by hiring people to clean or do yard work. Some couples rotate chores, or split things based on who has more time. Many of the mothers I interviewed had either cut back their hours at work or were staying home full time. Two of the fathers that I interviewed were home part time while also attending school.

Drs. Alexandra Sacks and Catherine Birndorf, authors of *What No One Tells You: A Guide to Your Emotions from Pregnancy to Motherhood*, advocate for discussing parenting roles. They use the terms *consciously* and *collaboratively* to describe how parents should approach taking on the task of divvying up parenting responsibilities. *Conscious* and *collaborative* basically describe how I want to make most of my parenting decisions and are in part what led me to write this book. *What No One Tells You* also introduced me to the concept of "supportive co-parenting," which is the style of parenting many millennial couples seem to be using these days. Gone are the assumptions that in a heterosexual couple the female partner will do all of the caregiving while the male partner is the sole income provider. The lines are way more blurry than that. Supportive co-parenting is more than just dividing the tasks to be done. It's supporting each other in the emotional experience of parenting, which is constant, challenging, and intense. Basically, you want to feel like you are on the same team with your partner. Otherwise it's you against everyone else, and that's not a great place to be.[22]

That last part is especially important to remember. On those long nights when I got up to feed the baby because, again, boobs, John would quietly whisper "You're a good mom" to me as I crawled exhaustedly back into bed. I felt so supported in that moment, and the resentment that may have been stewing about why I had to be the one to get out of bed yet again just because I was a freaking woman would dissolve. This can be challenging to navigate, especially for cisgender different-sex couples, given the centuries of baggage and very real societal standards that still exist today when it comes to our expectations of men and women. Same-sex couples might have it a little easier in this area without quite the same level of gender role bullshit to wade through when deciding who does what.

It is also important to keep in mind that just because you decide on something to begin with doesn't mean it is set in stone. Successful parenting is about being flexible and creative, and meeting your child where they are—which requires constant adaptation as new situations and challenges arise. This is what can make parenting creative and fun, and also make you want to pull out your hair. But it's a good reminder that if something is not working, you can change it. Adjust those schedules, try daycare, sleep in the guest room one night a week to get some peace. Do what works for you and your family. I promise no one is checking your video baby monitor feed to do a play-by-play on what goes on in your home. And it would be creepy AF if they were.

KNOW YOUR HISTORY

We know from the previous chapter that we all bring our histories with us into parenting. Part of that history is whatever roles we saw our parents take on growing up. This is important to note for a couple of reasons. First, we tend to fall into patterns that are familiar to us, so if we grew up in a household where the responsibilities were divided by heteronormative gender roles, then those will be our gut habits. We might assume that the female partner is going to do most of the childcare and household maintenance, and the male partner is going to do household repairs and lawncare. Second, it gives us background information for our partner's expectations. It can be helpful to know that your partner's mom always made lunch for him with a little note in it and that this was special to him—and that's why he pictures you doing it for your child. Or that your wife's dad was never around, so anytime you have to take a business trip she's going to experience not only the stress of parenting alone but also resurfaced feelings of abandonment and fear that your children will feel the same way. It can get messy quickly, and knowing our partner's history can help us put those situations into context and be more empathetic to their needs.

What Other Parents Said

I asked the parents I interviewed what roles they and their partner play in parenting, and how they divide responsibilities. Here is what they said:

MANAGER AND PLAYMATE

"Typically, I am the organizer and manager, while my husband is more of a playmate. However, we both stand firm on expectations and discipline."

"Since I am home full time, he tends to think I take care of everything with the kids, and he is the fun playtime dad. We are trying to make sure we are on the same page in helping him understand that even though you are at work all day we don't throw our structure out the window when you get home."

MOM AT HOME

"My wife does most of it since she is home full time, and when I come home, he wants to play. Whatever is happening in the evenings is what I do, like bath time and bedtime. We are both involved in parenting (depending on) whoever is home and there at the time."

"I have them during the day. He comes home and starts cooking, hits the ground running with them. We do a lot of divide and conquer. We are as fifty-fifty as we can be with me being at home full time. He does bath every night, and bedtime."

SHIFT WORK

"Ours is a very fluid household. Right now, my husband is in school and I take on more of the household responsibilities, but as for parenting we are on different schedules and it's rarely both of us with the kids. Usually one of us has them; we share equally in bedtime, school drop off, etc. I do most of the planning. Doctor's appointments, dentist, school events, homework due, etc., are all planned by me. He will show up when I tell him to."

"I am the primary parent five days out of the week. Two days a week my husband is home with her and is the primary parent. I take on most of the stuff with her, and I am her primary choice as well, so she comes to me more."

"We have similar roles, but our work schedules determine what we need to do at any given time. My wife works twelve-hour day shifts as a nurse, and she leaves before the children wake up, so when she gets home, they cling to her and I feel responsible for keeping them busy until she completes her post-work routine (changing, prepping for the next day of work, eating dinner, etc.). I work on the weekends at a church, so Saturdays and Sundays tend to keep her busy as the sole parent."

DAD AT HOME

"My husband is an amazing partner. When our daughter was very small, since I was exclusively breastfeeding, he was there with me for every feed. He would get me water and a snack or anything else I needed. He was also the exclusive diaper

changer for the first six weeks and overnight, since I was handling feeding. When our daughter was just over a year old, he changed jobs so that he could stay at home with her during the day while I worked. He is also the main cook and cleaner now that he's at home. A lot of times, he starts a task and I finish it. For example, he'll do laundry during the day and I'll fold it at night, or he'll cook dinner and I'll clean it up. I have always been the organizational center of the family, though he's getting better at that too. I pay the bills and make appointments and keep track of things."

DIVIDE AND CONQUER

"We both pretty much do everything at some point. When I was home full time, I was doing a lot during the day, and when he came home at night he would take over, do bath time, read stories, etc. He is probably more hands on when it comes to playing. I'm more of a 'go play by yourself while I clean the kitchen' parent. It just kind of happened. As time has gone on, and I worked for a few years and he had to step up, things got more even. With three kids we have to divide and conquer."

"We don't have traditional roles; he does all of the kitchen and I do the rest of the house. We trade off things without discussing it. It's just become second nature that we take turns."

"We divide responsibilities through verbal communication ('You get him ready for bed, and I'll get her ready'), by balancing each other's workload (i.e., 'I'll take care of as much as I can so my spouse and I can both focus on being a family when they get home'), or simply whichever of us is present when a need arises."

"I handle feeding our baby since I am breastfeeding. We both do a lot of getting him ready, picking out his clothes, bath time, etc. I do bedtime a lot of the time because I like to do

*it. My husband washes bottles and gets all of his stuff ready
in the mornings. Whoever is available to take care of it does
whatever needs to be done."*

FLUID ROLES

*"We switch back and forth between caregiver, disciplinarian,
and playmate. There are days I don't discipline well but my
husband is totally on it. And there are days he struggles to do
all the caretaker things and not feel overwhelmed. We each
try to get some sort of special time or playtime at least once
during the day."*

*"I would say we both wear many hats. My husband and I enjoy
playing and helping our daughter explore and learn, but we
both are also happy to put on our disciplinary hats and help our
daughter navigate the harder parts of her world."*

*"We're pretty fluid when it comes to responsibilities—it's a
case-by-case basis and I think we have a good ear for what's
needed from whom at any given moment. We also try to pay
attention to our own strengths and weaknesses. For instance,
I'm typically a night owl, so I tend to handle the kids if they
wake up before 3 a.m. and she tends to handle them after that.
Some things have just happened naturally. For whatever reason,
we started to notice that our three-year-old had trouble going
down for the night when my wife would do it, so I typically put
our three-year-old down."*

———

As you can see, we all do things a little bit differently. What
works for one family or child may not work for another. Don't
be afraid to experiment, try new things, and follow your
instincts. Generally, the worst-case scenario is that it doesn't

work, and you try something else. The key with all of this, like with most things in relationships, is communication. If you don't communicate it, your partner won't know about it. So, speak up, discuss your strategies, and express your needs. You are in this together pretty much for life, so get your team on the same page.

Practical Planning: Responsibilities

One thing to note up front for heterosexual couples is that like it or not, gender roles can be a deciding factor in the division of labor. A 2015 study by the Families and Work Institute found that when comparing same-sex couples to different-sex couples, the same-sex couples were more likely to divide household labor by personal preference or logic rather than gender roles. They were also more likely to share in childcare responsibilities.[23] This may or may not be your goal, depending on your relationship dynamics, and that is okay. Again, do what works for you. Either way, I recommend making a list of the tasks and responsibilities you think will be added to your plate after you become a parent, and then talk through that list together. Here is one to get you started:

- Feeding baby
- Changing diapers
- Giving baths
- Bedtime routine
- Laundry
- Nighttime wake-ups
- Making doctor's appointments
- Attending doctor's appointments
- Administering medication
- Washing bottles
- Playing with baby
- Preparing food
- Tidying
- Cleaning floors
- Taking out trash
- Grocery shopping

- Sorting and buying baby clothes
- Cleaning bathrooms
- Dusting
- Dishes
- Managing finances

This is not comprehensive, of course, but it should get your brain thinking about all of the things you will be sharing responsibility for. Once you have your list, you can go through each item and decide how you will handle it. Maybe mom or the partner who carried the baby plans to breast-feed, so dad or the non-carrying partner decides to handle all of the diapers at first. Maybe one of you is very particular about how laundry is done, so they should take that on. If dad is home a lot during the day, maybe mom does bath time each night to have special bonding time with baby in those few hours before bed and give dad a break. It can be whatever works for you, as long as it is conscious, communicated, and collaborative. What we are trying to avoid here is a sink full of ripe bottles and not a clean one in sight for the next feeding because both of you thought the other would wash them. Agreeing to this ahead of time also allows you to hold each other accountable. If you want to go so far as to write out the list and hang it on the fridge, go for it. It will probably make your life easier when trying to recall the details in the fog of sleep deprivation. The goal is for both of you to be in agreement regarding what you will take on, so that resentment doesn't build. Think of this as the first step in your practical communication about caring for your child. Practicing now gets you a head start for when you are in the trenches.

PAINT DONE

When discussing your tasks, you want to be clear on what completion for that task looks like. In her newest book, *Dare to Lead*, Brené Brown describes an exercise called "Paint Done" where you take a particular task and outline what "being done" looks like. What's the finished product? This is really asking "What expectations are behind this task for you?" I'll give you an example from my own house: baby laundry. If you asked John and me to describe "Paint Done" for baby laundry, you would get two different answers. I would say "Wash laundry with unscented detergent on normal with an extra rinse in the cycle and then dry on normal in the dryer without a dryer sheet. Fold, separating long-sleeve onesies, short-sleeve onesies, pants, pajamas, and rompers. Set aside any clothes that are too small and place them in the giveaway box. Sort folded clothes into their labeled dividers in the baby's room." John would say "Wash the clothes, dry without a dryer sheet, put away." See how they are different? I clearly have some very specific expectations for how I think baby laundry should be done. The "Paint Done" exercise brings those expectations to light so that you can then talk about how you want to handle it. In this situation, I might choose to do the laundry, since I am particular about how it's done. Or John might do it and I might have to adjust some of my expectations. Or we could divide it up, where John does the washing and drying, and I do the putting away. As long as we are on the same page and doing what works for us, we are good to go.

ALL SYSTEMS GO

Systems are a big tool for John and me in our household. We both tend to stick to responsibilities when they are a part of our routine and we both know what the expectations are. Although the systems have evolved according to our needs at the time, here are some we currently have in place:

- **You kill it you fill it.** This was a rule from our old camp days together. At mealtimes, if someone took the last of something, like juice, green beans, etc., they were responsible for filling it. We've applied this concept to our household. Paper towels, toilet paper, trash bags, cleaning supplies—if you kill it, you fill it. This is one of the systems that keeps our household running smoothly.

- **Daily pickup.** At the end of each day, we both spend time picking up various items off the floors of our house so that 1) the house stays tidy, and 2) our robot vacuum doesn't eat things. This daily reset keeps the clutter from creeping, for the most part.

- **Cleaning day.** Although we are pretty good at managing mess, the big cleaning tasks are harder for us to stay on top of. We schedule a cleaning day and tackle those things that aren't daily tasks, like bathrooms, mopping the floors, etc. We put this on the calendar so we are both committed to it, and we alternate who watches the kids and who cleans so we can both get our stuff done.

- **Alternate meals monthly.** We take turns monthly for who is in charge of meal planning and cooking. This is my favorite system we've implemented so far. I *love* not having to worry about what's for dinner for an entire month.

EMOTIONAL LABOR: SOMEONE'S GOT TO DO IT

What about the work that isn't generally itemized on a list? I'd like to add a few thoughts here on emotional labor—something John and I had already discussed early in our marriage. For those of you who are unfamiliar with the concept, *emotional labor* was coined by sociologist Arlie Hochschild in 1983 to describe the work that is involved in certain professions like therapists, pilots, nurses, customer service workers, and others whose jobs require them to manage or absorb some sort of heavy emotion.[24]

Today, the term has become a catch-all for work done by one partner (usually a woman in a different-sex relationship) that contributes to life management but largely goes unseen and undervalued. This could be mental labor, like keeping holiday gift lists in your head; actual emotional labor, such as managing your mother-in-law's feelings and keeping the family peace; or just regular labor, like making doctor's appointments or doing household chores. When a child arrives, it is often the woman who takes on the lion's share of these responsibilities, adding to what she already has to do at home and at work. Although modern millennial dads are doing more than ever before, a 2019 *Atlantic* article revealed that married American women spend twice as much time on housework and childcare as their male counterparts. They also spend more time today on childcare than mothers did in the 1960s, whether they are working or not.[25] That's a big gap.

Erica Djossa, a therapist whose *Happy as a Mother* community has a large online following, writes a popular Instagram series titled "The Invisible Load of Motherhood." This is the best illustration of emotional labor I've seen. She features a different domestic chore for each edition and highlights all the aspects of emotional labor that go into that one task. For example, in the "mealtime" edition, she lists things like:

- Deciding what to make
- Making sure you have all of the groceries
- Being mindful of budget

- Considering preferences
- Cleaning dishes

In an edition on bottle feeding, she lists:

- Cleaning and sterilizing all the things
- Finding the right formula and bottle
- Thinking ahead to make sure you don't run out
- The cost of formula
- Dealing with unwanted "Breast Is Best" comments

It's not just the act of giving a baby a bottle. It's everything that feeds into that (pun intended). Erica really breaks down those parenting tasks into all of the mental, emotional, and physical aspects, and brings to life the emotional labor that is so often hidden in the background but is as important—and draining—as any other chore.

Practical Planning: Childcare and Career Changes

Now is the time to do some general practical planning around leave from work, any job adjustments that need to be made, and plans for childcare. John and I both worked full-time before we had our daughter, and we both wanted to continue working after she was born. I was able to take twelve weeks' leave from my job, and John could take two. We made the decision to both be home during the first two weeks after our baby arrived as we tried to figure out how to care for a newborn for the first time and as I was physically recovering from birth. We decided that when my twelve weeks' leave was up, we would hire a part-time nanny to provide childcare while we both worked. This felt like the best fit for us since we only needed someone about three days a week, we could afford it, and we liked the idea of our child developing a special bond with this person.

There were other practical concerns to discuss as well, such as creating a will after our daughter was born. We also talked about who her guardians might be in the event that something happened to us, and we spoke with those people to make sure they were comfortable committing to that role. We drew up nearly all of our will before the birth so that afterward we just had to fill in her information before finalizing it. We also decided some fun things, like who to choose as our daughter's godparents, and if and when we wanted to have her baptized, which is a huge tradition in my family. Again, I was glad we had these conversations early and decided most of these things before our child arrived. I didn't want to be arguing the merits of daycare versus nanny when I was exhausted, frustrated, and feeling stir crazy during those weeks of maternity leave.

Lastly, I want to reiterate that even if you decide these things ahead of time, they are not set in stone. As we have already established, babies bring nothing but change. I was open to the possibility that I might not want to go back to work, and John and I addressed what that might look like ahead of time, in case it came up later. (It didn't. I am definitely a person who needs to work for my own mental health.) Our child could have had a medical issue that required us to take more time off of work to care for her. We could have changed our minds about childcare, or who her guardians would be. All of that is perfectly normal. Children and families are not stagnant. They are ever-evolving, and these are not necessarily "one and done" decisions. Give yourself permission to change your mind if something doesn't feel like it fits anymore. The most important thing to do is to keep that line of communication open with your partner.

Summary

- Discussing your parenting roles with your partner ahead of time can help set expectations and avoid conflict down the road when you are sleep-deprived and stressed.

- The goal in discussing roles is to know what your responsibilities are ahead of time, and to avoid tasks falling through the cracks because you both assumed the other would do it. The goal is also for both you and your partner to be in agreement about what each of you will take on, so that resentment doesn't build.

- Gender roles, expectations, schedules, and your current household division of labor all factor into these discussions and how work is divided.

- These decisions aren't set in stone. If something isn't working, adjust it.

- Remember to be flexible. Give yourself and your partner permission to change your mind if something doesn't feel like it fits anymore. The most important thing to do is to keep that line of communication open.

Discussion Topics:
Roles

1. What roles did each of your parents take on when you were children?

2. Make a list of all of the tasks you think you will have after you bring your baby home, and then decide who will do what.

3. What systems can you implement at home that will limit conflict about domestic chores?

4. How long will each of you be at home after your baby is born or your adopted child comes home?

5. Do you want to stagger parental leave, or take it together?

6. Will either of you stay home full-time or part-time? Or will you both go back to work?

7. What is your childcare plan? Daycare? Nanny? Family member?

8. What is your plan for when your child has a sick day or childcare falls through?

Determining Your Discipline and Parenting Style

"Having children is like living in a frat house—nobody sleeps, everything's broken, and there's a lot of throwing up."

—RAY ROMANO

I WOULDN'T BE SURPRISED if you read the title of this chapter and thought, *Seriously, Lindsay? We don't even have a baby yet, and you want us to talk about discipline? Isn't that putting the cart before the horse?* I don't think so. First, by now you know I am an overplanning weirdo who likes to have her ducks in a row—and thinks you should too. And secondly, determining discipline and how you will parent is much deeper, bigger, and more important than just correcting your child when they do something wrong. It reflects your family's core values and practices. It comprises your and your partner's histories and how you apply them to parenting. It affects the skills, behaviors, values, and characteristics you choose to instill in your children. When I use the term *discipline* I'm not just talking about how you will "punish" your kids when they misbehave. I'm using this word as an umbrella term that encompasses your guiding parenting philosophy and strategy. This starts even before your child is born and drives so many decisions you make as a parent. It is the first step in thinking intentionally about how you want to manage boundaries, teach your children values that are important to you, and shape your relationship with your child.

One Size Does Not Fit All

I think we all sometimes wish there were a "one-size-fits-all" approach to discipline and parenting. Sort of like Ikea instructions where if we just follow the illustrated steps we'll end up with a reasonably stable structure. We want to do the right thing and have it turn out okay. The good news and bad news is that parenting and discipline styles are never uniform, and each child and situation necessitate different strategies. For me, this is one of the things that makes parenting fun. It is a never-ending puzzle to navigate and figure out. Although challenging, those times where you fit the pieces together and it works are moments of great joy.

I want to illustrate this principle by sharing this scene from when my daughter was seven months old and just getting the hang of crawling. She spies a toy across the room that she wants, and laboriously makes her way toward it. I sit nearby, watching her struggle and work her way toward her goal. She isn't upset, but she's clearly working hard. Her little baby grunts are tiny versions of a weightlifter straining for one more rep. I am positively itching to help. The toy is within arm's reach. It would be so easy to just hand it to her. *She's worked enough*, I think. *I'm just going to help her out.* But *No*, the voice in the back of my head says. *Remember, she can do this. And she will learn through practice, and trying, and struggling.* So, I sit back. I fight the urge to get the toy, and I watch as approximately one million hours later she finally reaches her fat little hand out and grabs it. The joy on her face is infectious. She is preening with pride at her accomplishment. And you know what? So am I.

Giving my child space to figure things out on her own is part of my parenting philosophy, which I would characterize as one of observation and curiosity. When my toddler is exploring, I watch her to see what she is looking for, if she seems to have an end goal as she climbs on a rock, if she can physically handle it, and what I might need to do to support her in her exploration. When she is having a total meltdown right before naptime, I tend to let it go, associating it with being tired. This is generally how I approach parenting. Although the strategies may change depending on age and needs, the general framework of curiosity, observation, and support will likely be consistent for me. Why? Because I've thought about it, and that's the type of parent I deliberately strive to be.

Parenting Styles

Let's dig a little deeper into what factors influence our parenting styles. One of the most common factors that determine how we parent is *doing what we know*—meaning we defer to what our parents did. For example, there are many ways in which I parent that mirror what my mom did, such as:

- I generally give my child more time for free play than a lot of parents I know.
- I encourage independence and exploration.

- I believe in letting kids be bored.
- I try to play a lot of games.
- I also try to have my child be outside as much as possible.

These are all things I experienced when I was growing up, and I look back on them fondly. Curious to see if other parents did the same, I asked my interviewees what things they do—positive or negative—that echo what their parents did. I got a variety of answers:

"I cook like my mom, almost every night. I make that a priority, showing my love for food."

"I catch myself having high expectations for my kids like my parents did, and I have to watch myself sometimes to make those reasonable and not push him past what is appropriate."

"Asking for respect. My mom demanded respect. I find myself telling my oldest not to be rude and to be respectful, and then I think, I sound just like my mom."

"My parents were so great about following our lead and being interested in what we wanted to be interested in, and they never shaped us. With mine it is the most fun to figure out what he likes and just follow it."

"The 'mom eyes.' My mom could give a look and that was all it really took. My gut reaction is I will do that and use a really stern voice and my daughter does not like that. She asks me, 'Why are you using a mean voice?'"

"I say 'I love you' a lot like my dad did."

———

We likely all have moments where we open our mouths and our mom or dad comes out. This became abundantly clear to me one evening when our daughter was a few months old, and John and I were doing the usual bedtime routine with her. We were attempting to wrestle her chubby arms out of her onesie and into pajamas. I raised my arms above my head to get her to mimic me, and cheerfully urged, "Skin the rabbit!" I didn't think about this; it just came out of my mouth as a reflex. A few minutes later, John stopped and asked, "What did you just say?" I repeated it. He looked at me like I was insane, and asked, "What does that even mean?" I explained that it meant to lift your arms above your head so that you could peel a shirt off. And then I thought about it more . . . peeling a shirt off . . . you know, like you would *peel the skin off a dead rabbit* after you killed it. Holy shit. That is *not* the visual I want to use in reference to my baby! Also, gross. We laughed about it together, and John asked me where that phrase had come from. I said I wasn't sure; my mom had always used it when I was a kid. A couple of days later my mom and I were chatting on the phone and I asked her where the phrase came from. She said *she* didn't know. Her mother just always said it to her. So here I was referencing skinning a dead animal when trying to dress my precious baby just because someone had done it before me, and I had never really thought about it.

How many of us do this all the time? We learn something at work that our manager taught us, never questioning whether it is the best way to do it. We argue with our partners about how to "correctly" fold a towel, when each of our correct ways are just the way we did it growing up. We push our kids to be independent because that's what our parents did, and we like that quality in ourselves. We spank them because we got spanked and feel like we turned out fine. But what if we took the time to pause and reflect on those things we do "just because" and decide if they work for us and for our child?

As Drs. Daniel J. Siegel and Tina Payne Bryson say in their book *The Power of Showing Up*, "History is not destiny."[26] Repeat that to yourself if you need to. History is *not* destiny. You have the power to harness your own history and change the way you parent. Humans are wonderfully adaptable. We aren't stuck in one place. But change takes effort, and self-awareness, and digging deep, which can be really hard for some of us, especially if what we uncover is painful.

This is an especially important point to consider when it comes to determining how you will discipline your child. When I asked the parents I interviewed, it didn't surprise me that most of them hadn't discussed discipline before having kids. After all, when you are planning for a newborn, it seems like one of those things you won't have to deal with for a while, and so many other matters take priority. Among those who did discuss it, many weighed the issue of whether or not to spank their child. Most of these parents were spanked as children and didn't want to do the same with their kids. It appears there is a generational shift happening when it comes to spanking. Speaking of which . . .

A Note about Spanking

Please allow me a soapbox about spanking. I know it is a heated topic, and that you might disagree with me. But I would be remiss if I did not take this opportunity to speak about an issue that I feel strongly about. I promise I will try to keep it brief.

As I am sure you may have guessed by now, I do not advocate for spanking as a discipline strategy. My best argument for this is that the research says it isn't effective, that it doesn't lead to real behavior change or learning, and that it can be detrimental to a child's brain development. In their book *No-Drama Discipline*, Siegel and Bryson explain that spanking (and really any form of fear-based discipline) is counterproductive to the goals of changing behavior and building a child's brain. A child's brain is unable to process that their safe person, who is supposed to protect them when they are scared or in pain, is also the one *causing* fear or pain. Spanking also teaches children that one way to resolve conflict is to inflict physical pain on another person.[27] My more judgmental argument is that I just think it's uncreative parenting. We've evolved so far from the "spare the rod, spoil the child" mentality that most parents I know do not utilize physical discipline as their primary mode of punishment. Those I talked to who do use it say they keep it in their repertoire as a "last resort," or that "it's the only thing that works when nothing else does." Here's what this tells me. Using spanking as a "last resort" implies that you have tried everything else you've thought of and none of it is working; this indicates that you are not using spanking with intention and to teach. It also tells me that you are likely spanking your child when you are angry or frustrated, which any parent would understandably be if they have exhausted all of their options in the moment and don't know what to do. Imagine how scary that would be for your child. On a podcast called *Totally Mommy*, the host Elizabeth Laime often makes the argument against spanking by comparing it to domestic violence. In our country, if you hit your spouse or partner, it is socially and legally unacceptable. Why, then, do we condone hitting our children, an arguably weaker and more vulnerable little person who is just trying to figure out how the world works? It makes no sense. Okay, stepping down off my soapbox now. I did enjoy the extra height for a few minutes.

Choosing Your Discipline Strategies

When I asked parents what influenced their discipline strategy decisions, the sources narrowed down into just a few categories:

1. What their own parents did when they were growing up.
2. What other people they know do or did (siblings, friends, etc.).
3. What books or other research says to do.
4. Trial and error.

I want to be clear about something: Whatever the source of our strategies, we are all going to do number four. Trial and error is pretty much the only way to figure out what works and what doesn't with your particular child. It's why so many people say you can't truly understand what it is like to be a parent until you are one. It's a hands-on learning experience. Based on this fact, I think it is a good idea to explore all of these things and see which resonates with you and your partner. Did you like what your parents did? Or was it terrible for you? Start to notice how friends interact with their kids or watch your nieces and nephews at family gatherings and explore your reactions. Maybe read a book or two (see the Resources section for recommendations). From there, you should have a good pool of strategies to start experimenting with when the time comes, and hopefully have some boundaries in place about what is okay and what is not okay for your family.

I want to be very clear that when it comes to choosing discipline strategies and exploring how you want to raise your children, you need to focus on what works for *your* family. Just because someone else does it one way, or some expert says to do it another way, doesn't mean it will be right for you and your child. Brainstorm, explore, get ideas from other sources, but at the end of the day, stay true to what your family and your child needs.

Shark Music

I strongly urge you to think about discipline now, because one day, sooner or later, when you are least expecting it, you are going to hear "shark music" when interacting with your child. Let me explain. Shark music, a concept created by parenting organization Circle of Security International, happens when some interaction with your child triggers a fear reaction in you as a parent. One thing that does it for me is when my child makes a mess. It might be a mess in play or it might be an accidental spill, but I feel anger rise involuntarily and immediately. I haven't been able to directly connect this to something I experienced as a child just yet, but I've noticed the pattern and have been focusing on recognizing and managing it when it comes up. The shark music moments might be subconsciously connected to something that happened to you when you were young, or it might come from an experience where your child got hurt or something frightening happened. It is called "shark music" after the ominous theme from *Jaws* that played every time the shark was about to attack.

You know you are experiencing shark music when your heart beats faster, your breath gets shallower, you start sweating, or your face gets hot. It is important to be aware of what causes shark music for us as parents because often it is a false alarm. If we parent from a place of fear, we aren't being intentional, and we are letting our own primitive brains hijack us and our interactions with our children.[28] We might experience shark music when something from our attachment history is triggered, such as if our parents got upset or we were punished when we made a mess, had a meltdown in public, or lied about something. We might experience it when we encounter a situation with our child that was scary to us when we were kids. Or maybe we are just overwhelmed and don't know what we are doing, so our shark music is the background soundtrack of our perpetually exhausted parent brain. Either way, this is important to be aware of. Why? Because when we experience shark music, we don't parent with intention. We are likely just having gut reactions. Let's go back to my mess example: If my child spills a cup of water, even if it is a total accident, my gut reaction is anger and disappointment. It may be that I experienced anger or disappointment from an adult as a child when I made a mess, and that's why those feeling come up for me. Regardless, the reaction doesn't match the situation; it is much more intense. I've had to learn to notice this reaction and intentionally respond with kindness and calm in the moment, when my gut really wants to say "Seriously, kid?! Now I have to clean up this mess!" Most people don't make the best decisions when we are in a place of fear. Our brains aren't wired that way. When we experience shark music, it is important that we learn to recognize and manage it so it doesn't hijack our parenting. How do we do this? By taking steps to parent in an intentional—not reactive—way. There are a few key steps to doing this:

1. We can parent more intentionally by proactively taking care of ourselves (more about self-care in chapter 10). We are much more vulnerable to shark music when we are tired, hungry, overwhelmed, or experiencing strong emotions.

2. We learn to recognize when shark music is happening, which means paying attention to how our brains and bodies are reacting in particular situations. You can spot

this if you are getting all riled up about a specific behavior or scenario with your child, and your partner isn't. This is usually a good sign that something is being triggered that is specific to you. Once you find yourself able to recognize when your shark music is playing, you can practice calming your body down when it happens. This might mean removing yourself from the situation if you can and coming back when you are calmer. I can generally calm myself down by taking some deep breaths wherever I am at that moment. Find what works for you and practice it when your shark music starts blaring.

3. We reflect on how we handled certain situations. We know that no parent is perfect, which means we are going to mess things up. Going back and thinking about what happened, what triggered us, how we reacted, and how we could have handled things differently will help us the next time it happens. Reflection is how we improve as people and as parents.

4. Finally, we go back and repair with our child if needed. We apologize for yelling, or leaving, or whatever we did that severed connection with our child. We talk about what we plan to do next time. This not only repairs the relationship, but it models for our child how to manage it when they mess up. The research shows that secure attachment is only 30 percent getting things right. The other 70 percent is about repairing things when we mess up.[29]

Is intentional parenting really that important? I think so. Scientific research shows that *repeated experiences actually change our child's brain.* When we experience something over and over again, this creates a neural pathway in the brain specific to that experience. For example, when we are learning something new, such as how to play an instrument, we have to practice and practice, but eventually our brain learns how to do it, and we can even do it without thinking about it too much if the connection is strong enough. The more the experience is repeated, the stronger the neural pathway. The same goes for our children. Let that sink in.[30] If we give our child food and give them ownership over what they eat and when their body tells them they are full, their brain will build neural pathways for listening to their body and gauging when they are full. If, however, we dictate how much or what they have to eat or insist that they clean their plate at every meal, their brain will build neural pathways for shutting down that "full" response and focus instead on clearing their plate to please us. As a result, they may not have the ability to connect to the sensation of feeling "full" in their body. That is powerful stuff. As parents, you have the awesome ability to choose how you want to shape those connections.

Mission Possible: Creating a Mission Statement

A couple of years ago I went to a training session on trauma with Marshall Lyles, a well-known play therapist and adoptive parent. The training was designed for parents whose children have a history of trauma and the professionals who support their families. One of the key points Lyles made was to compare the focus on short-term goals and long-term goals when dealing with and disciplining children. When we focus on short-term goals in our children, he explained, we tend to zero in more on compliance and survival, basically just reacting to whatever we experience in the moment.

When we concentrate on long-term goals, we can see the bigger picture of a situation or behavior, and are more likely to intentionally respond rather than react. Having a long-term goal of, for example, *emotional intelligence* helps us decide in the moment what is important.

Let's put this into practice. If my child is having a big feeling, I am first going to choose to support her in expressing and naming that feeling, and only then discuss the behavior that came out of the big feeling, like throwing a toy across the room. This doesn't mean I don't address the behavior; it just helps me prioritize what to focus on with my child to build the skills I want her to have. In a nutshell, you can elect to do what is easy now and play the short game, or you can choose what might be harder now but will make it easier in the future and play the long game. Most parents don't even get the opportunity to think about this before they are drowning in spit-up, diapers, and sleepless nights. To help parents think more deeply about their short-term and long-term goals for parenting, Marshall suggests creating a parenting mission statement to help guide decisions. The mission statement exercise accomplishes two things, Marshall asserts: the first is to create intention in parenting by stating what our purpose with our children is, and the second is to shift the focus from the short-term goals of daily compliance and survival to the long-term goals of raising well-adjusted young adults.

I attended this training when my daughter had just turned one. Here's what I came up with as a mission statement to guide my long-term focus in parenting:

> *To be the best guide for my child as she*
> *discovers who she is, what she loves, and*
> *how to become a functioning adult.*

I shared this with John after the training, since he wasn't able to attend, and he agreed with what I had written. About a year later, I would say this still fits. When I interact with my two-year-old, we are focused on exploring and learning. I don't try to direct her play, but I do try to point out things that she might love to discover, like the fuzzy caterpillar on the ground, or how you can see a rainbow in a puddle sometimes. I am her guide, yes, but not her dictator. I want to leave her space to figure things out on her own, to fall in love with interests that may be different from ours, and to support her in those pursuits. So, while the parenting mission statement can guide us long-term, it doesn't have to be fixed. I imagine mine might change as our daughter gets older, or as we decide to focus on different things. The point is not so much to adhere to it to the letter; rather, it is to thoughtfully and intentionally consider what direction you are going in, and to use your long-term parenting goals to guide day-to-day decisions.

There's another area where your mission statement will come in handy. The moment we enter the parenting game (and this can start as early as when you are trying to get pregnant), people offer unsolicited advice on everything from conceiving to whether you should want a boy or a girl to opinions about staying home full-time. All of that before your kid even gets here! This doesn't even factor in the all-encompassing comparison trap of social media, which can be never-ending. Your mission statement can be your guidepost when the voices of the peanut gallery intrude. It is your lighthouse, your safe haven, your rock to return to again and again whenever you find yourself questioning your parenting decisions.

Your mission statement should include two parts: 1) An all-encompassing statement that gives a theme for how you plan to parent; and 2) a short list of things that are important to your family when it comes to parenting. This second part is a wonderful trick taken from the world of wedding planning. In her book *A Practical Wedding,* author Meg Keene instructs couples to choose the things about their wedding that are most important to them and let go of the rest. Maybe they choose the photographer and the food. That means they take a stand on and set strong boundaries for those two things and show more flexibility on or let go of everything else.[31] Although I will admit the stakes are higher when it comes to our children, you can apply a similar strategy here. I'll use myself as an example to illustrate. You will remember my parenting mission statement from earlier in the chapter: *"To be the best guide for my child as she discovers who she is, what she loves, and how to become a functioning adult."*

That's my overall approach right now, and here are the particular aspects I've chosen to focus on:

1. **Encouraging independent exploration and play:** We want our daughter to follow her interests, so most of the time we let her lead in play. We also want her to learn to use her imagination and learn to play on her own and with other children, so we have a lot of open-ended toys and books in our home, and we spend a lot of time outside.

2. **Developing life skills:** Our toddler has things she is responsible for at home, like taking her plate to the sink when she is done eating, helping unload the dishwasher, and putting her toys away. Now that she is more verbal, we practice polite phrases, like saying *please* and *thank you.* We also focus on emotional regulation as a life skill, talking about feelings, helping her name and learn about them, and incorporating a lot of social skills lessons from

Daniel Tiger, the cartoon descendent of *Mister Rogers' Neighborhood* that has a jingle for just about every life situation a preschooler might find themselves in.

3. **Developing identity:** We want to let our daughter learn who she is and grow into the person she is meant to be. This means we don't impose a lot of stereotypes or expectations on her. We have been intentional about having a variety of toys, not just ones for "girls," and exposing her to different worlds and interests through books.

4. **Having healthy sleep habits:** If I don't sleep, I am my worst self as a parent. I extend this to my daughter as well. We have strong boundaries around routines, nap times, and bedtimes, and for the most part don't deviate from them.

In creating the mission statement, I factored in our long-term hopes for our child (remember those from chapter 4?). My main hope was that my children have success in their lives, whatever that looks like for them. Our mission statement reflects *what* we want to do to guide our child, and the more specific values below indicate *how* we plan to reach that bigger goal. Will they evolve as our child grows? Totally. But they are the guidepost we use when we are trying to decide if something is worth worrying about. If it isn't on the list, we have to decide, *Do we let this go, or is it something we want to add?* I caution you: Keep this list short. Under five items if you can.

Choose Your Battles

As a parent and a human, you don't have the ability to go to the mat on every single matter when it comes to your child. Trust me, you will burn out faster than you can say

"Daniel Tiger's Neighborhood." That's the entire point of this exercise—to give yourself guidance on where you want to expend your energy and time, and what you can let go of. One of the stock phrases you hear parents say when it comes to discipline is "choose your battles." But what does that mean? If you have outlined your mission statement and family values, then choosing your battles means deciding what is important enough to take a stand on, and where you can be more flexible.

Going back to my example, you will notice there isn't anything about food on my list. This is an area I have chosen to be more flexible on. It doesn't mean I don't care about it and that I let my child eat cookies for every meal. But it does mean I don't put a lot of stock in it if my child chooses not to eat something. It means I don't spend a ton of time thinking about it and planning for it. I am not going to enter a power struggle with my child over her taking three more bites of chicken, because that is not where I want to put my energy. It's something I can be more flexible on, because it isn't on my list of top priorities right now, and I am okay with that.

Values, Simplified

If creating a mission statement feels overwhelming, let's try something more basic: Choose one or two values to use as a framework for your parenting style. Defining values gives you a filter to run things through, and helps you identify what is important to you in parenting and in life. The easiest way I've found to choose values is to look at a list of them, reflect on each value, and then choose the ones that fit for you. The trick is to not choose too many. These should be "umbrella" words that other things can fall under—not every single thing you care about. Here's a sampling:

- Accomplishment
- Adventure
- Capability
- Comfort
- Competence
- Cooperation
- Creativity
- Decisiveness
- Dependability
- Determination
- Discovery
- Empathy
- Excellence
- Expertise
- Faith
- Fitness
- Genuineness
- Growth
- Harmony
- Helpfulness
- Honesty
- Integrity
- Intuition
- Joy
- Kindness
- Leadership
- Loyalty
- Open-mindedness
- Passion
- Playfulness
- Presence
- Reflection
- Reliability
- Sensitivity
- Service
- Stability
- Teamwork
- Thrift
- Trust
- Warmth
- Wisdom
- Zeal

This is just a start. If you'd like to see a longer list, look up "list of value words" online and you'll get hundreds. Reflect on these and circle the ones that speak to you. Try for five or less at first. Once you have those, let them simmer for a bit. Then come back and try to narrow it down to two or three. When I did this exercise, I started off marking *competence*, *creativity*, *integrity*, and *reliability*. After reflecting on those words, I narrowed it down to two: *integrity* and *creativity*. Then I defined what those words meant for me.

Integrity:

- Choosing what is right over what is easy
- Sticking to my word

Creativity:

- Being curious and following my whims
- Exploring new ideas and inspiration

I use these two values in my day-to-day life to help steer me, but I also use them in my parenting. I choose to teach my child new skills and set boundaries rather than giving in because it is easier in the moment. I try my best to follow through when I say I will do something. I am at the top of my game as a parent when I am being creative, making up a new game, singing and dancing, or thinking through new approaches to a challenging behavior. My values are a guidepost for me. If I am not living these things, then I know something is off. My plate is too full; I am overwhelmed; I am letting what I should do get in the way of what I know is right for me. When that happens, it's my sign to course correct and do what I can to get back to those basic values.

Triggers and Repairs

We've established that we all have our own attachment history that influences how we parent, and that our specific shark music can pop up when we get triggered. Now let's talk about what those triggers might look like, and how we can fix things when we inevitably make a mistake or lose our cool with our child. I asked the parents I interviewed what behaviors or situations with their kids were triggers for them, and here is a list of some of the things they said:

- Not listening
- Outright defiance
- Whining
- Rebelling
- Getting upset easily
- Eye rolls
- Meltdowns over something minor
- Lying
- When I feel disrespected
- Talking back
- When everything is messy
- Power struggles
- Not sleeping
- Screaming

Sounds fun, right? The reality is, we are all going to lose patience with our child at some point or another. It might be tied to something from our own history, or we might just be exhausted and spread too thin, which makes us even more vulnerable to our shark music. It happens to every parent. So, what do we do when this happens? Feel guilty? Beat ourselves up about it? Blame our child to avoid facing our own stuff? Hopefully not. Research has found that in those moments where we flip our lids as parents, if we can go back and repair the disconnection with our child, we end up even more connected than we were before. In fact, a scientist named Edward Tronick found that in his observations of parents and their child, "miscoordination" happened 70 percent of the time. Seventy percent! That means that parents were only getting it right 30 percent of the time. Tronick found that those parents who noticed the disconnection in that 70 percent window and made attempts to repair had children who were securely attached.[32] So not only do you not have to get it right all the time, when you do mess up it actually becomes an opportunity for greater connection with your child *if* you go back and repair the relationship.

Here's what I mean by "repair." Imagine if every time you had a disagreement or were hurtful to your spouse, partner, or best friend you did not go back and resolve it. Say you called your partner lazy for not pitching in more around the house. Or your best friend bailed on dinner plans at the last minute and didn't apologize. Maybe your spouse threw away your favorite ratty old T-shirt from high school because they thought it was trash. How would that affect your relationship? For most of us, it wouldn't be good, and would likely erode our connection over time. To prevent this, we have to go back and repair. We apologize for the hurtful thing we said. Perhaps we say, "You aren't lazy; I am sorry I said that. I am just feeling overwhelmed and frustrated," or "I think I have too much on my plate with the household tasks I am doing currently. Can we talk about how to shift some things so I feel less overwhelmed?" Sometimes it is a simple apology, and sometimes it might be a deeper conversation around problem-solving or processing emotions. Either way, you tackle the problem as a team instead of letting it be a wedge between you. The same happens with our children. The end goal is reconnection.

———

We've talked about a lot of intense and deep stuff in this chapter, so let's end with a little parenting pep talk. Please know you are already an intentional parent; the fact that you care enough to read this book and prepare for your child's arrival proves it. Your willingness to explore your own history and what you bring to the table as a mom or dad will only benefit your child and deepen your relationship with them. You have the ability to choose how you want to teach your child and determine the values you want to focus on. Only you can decide what is important for you. You know your child and your family best. You've got this.

Summary

- Your discipline strategy is much deeper, bigger, and more important than just correcting your child when they do something wrong. It is the first step in thinking intentionally about how you want to manage boundaries, teach your children values that are important to you, and shape your relationship with your child.

- Shark music happens when an interaction with our child triggers a fear reaction in us as parents. This might be subconsciously connected to something that happened to us when we were young, or it might stem from an experience where our child got hurt or something frightening happened.

- We bring our attachment histories and potential shark music triggers to the table when we parent. If we can identify these challenges going in, we can be more self-aware and more intentional in how we respond to our children.

- When it comes to the parenting mission statement, choosing discipline strategies, and exploring how you want to raise your children, you need to focus on what works for *your* family. Trust your gut before you poll every parent on Facebook.

- Identifying your parenting mission statement and areas of focus gives you a guide for what is important for your family and your child and allows you to let go of or be more flexible on things that aren't.

- The reality is we are all going to lose patience with our child at some point or another. Research has found that in those moments when we flip our lids as parents, if we can go back and repair the disconnection with our child, we end up even more connected than before.

- Your willingness to explore your own history and what you bring to the table as a mom or dad will only benefit your child and deepen your relationship with them. You have the ability to choose how you want to teach your child and what values you want to instill.

Discussion Topics:
Discipline

1. How were each of you disciplined as a child?

2. What shark music might you bring with you to parenting? What do you think your triggers will be?

3. What is something your mom or dad did when you were a kid that you think you might do as a parent? (This can be positive or negative.)

4. What discipline strategies do you think you might use with your future child?

5. Write a parenting mission statement.

6. Choose up to five values reflected in your mission statement to focus on in day-to-day parenting.

Villages and Boundaries

"Boundaries mean 'I am going to love you and love myself at the same time.'"

—CLEO WADE

GREW UP WITH a huge extended Catholic family, most of whom lived in Fort Worth, Texas. We saw each other at church on Sundays, had large family celebrations on almost every holiday, and spent countless days at my great-grandparents' house playing in the backyard. I had a pack of cousins with whom I went fishing, had sleepovers, and generally ran around for most of my childhood. I had always pictured my children having a similar experience. Gaggles of family; kids to play outside and get dirty with; a huge cheering section at every sporting event, recital, or graduation. But then John and I moved four hours away. Initially, our goal was to delay having a child until we could get back to Fort Worth, but we didn't know when that would happen. It could be five years; it could be ten. And it wasn't realistic to put our lives on hold in that way. Once we did become pregnant, I became less concerned about my child having cousins to play with and way more worried about how the hell I was going to care for a baby without the support of my family nearby.

My mom and I have a *Gilmore Girls*, us-against-the-world-style relationship, except with some clearer parental roles and healthier boundaries, and her wife has known me since I was a child. John has positive relationships with both of his parents and stepparents. While we didn't know how available their in-person support would be living four hours away, we knew we could count on them for emotional support. Since our daughter was the first grandchild on both sides of our families, everyone was *very* interested in being involved. We gave updates on doctor's appointments, shared when we chose a name, and attended baby showers lovingly thrown by family and friends. Our support system, though removed, was engaged months before our child ever arrived. I also sought out a therapist during this time, as I wanted to find someone who could guide me through the fears and anxieties of pregnancy, birth, and new motherhood, and someone we could also see as a couple if needed.

Ask for What You Need

A few months before our daughter was born, John and I both had discussions with our families about how they could support us in those early days of parenting. We ended up having shifts of family members at our house for about a month after the baby came. First my mom and stepmom, then John's mom, and finally my sister-in-law. Although it was sometimes overwhelming to have someone else in our space and home during that initial transition, the trade-off of the support and help that we got was definitely worth it. Our family was so great at focusing on what would help us as parents and not just cuddling a baby, or worse, expecting to be entertained while we tried to attend to our newborn's every need. I realize that a lot of this comes from being a part of families with healthy relationships and boundaries, but we also did some intentional setting of expectations leading up to this time.

Below is an email that we sent out to family members about a month before our daughter was born:

Hello Dear Family,

As the time approaches for our baby to arrive, we thought it would be a good idea to send out some information to those of you who will be visiting soon after she comes. Below is a list of things to keep in mind, and some attachments you may find useful.

Phone Tree: We have created a phone tree (attached) for when baby arrives to help spread the news. Please take a look at it so that you know who you may be calling. We respectfully ask that you do not post anything on social media until we have made an announcement.

Visiting Plan: All of our visitors have pretty flexible schedules. We have talked with each of you about your preferences, length of stay, etc., in general, but of course nothing can really be planned until the baby comes. **John will be the point person for coordinating visitors**, so plan to be in touch with him after our little one arrives.

Things to keep in mind when visiting:

- While we are going to be overjoyed at our baby girl's arrival, and we know you are too, please remember that visitors within the first month or two are there primarily to support us as parents. See "ways you can help" below.
- As part of supporting us as new parents, we ask you to give us space during your visit to get our footing and bond with the baby. We will of course desperately beg for help if we need it but want to have the opportunity to get our new parent sea legs. As most of you have been in our shoes, we are sure you remember what those first few months were like.

- If you are staying in our home, please prepare to keep yourselves entertained while you are here. Our focus is going to be on the baby, not on playing hosts.
- Lindsay is planning to breastfeed, so there will be various levels of nudity happening, especially in those first few weeks as both she and baby are getting the hang of things together. Don't say we didn't warn you. :)

Ways you can help:

- Offer encouragement to us in our rookie attempts at keeping a tiny human alive.
- Bring or cook us food.
- Do a task around the house (see attached list for some suggestions; there is also a copy that will be on our fridge).
- If someone asks how they can support us, recommend that they send a meal, or a gift card to a local restaurant (attached is a list of places that will deliver to us, and what we like to eat there).
- Give us grace, as we will be overwhelmed, and sleep deprived.

Thank you all for your support, love, and celebration on our journey so far. We are so grateful to have you as our village and are so excited for you to meet this precious girl when she decides to grace us with her presence. :)

Love to you all,
Lindsay and John

Was this excessive? Probably. Did it help me feel more in control going into this time? Definitely. Did our family and friends respect our boundaries and expectations? For the most part, yes. We were reasonably sure that if we communicated what we needed, our people would see and respect that. We also have the type of relationships where if something isn't working, we can have a conversation about it. I only had one meltdown during this time, which led to John awkwardly hugging me in our bedroom while I sobbed that I just wanted my house back to myself and that I was worried that having this meltdown with our napping newborn strapped to me would bathe her in stress hormones and *what if I was ruining her for life?*

My point in sharing all of this with you is to convey that to some extent, you can plan for this time. First, identify who can support you. You know your people best. You might have family or friends nearby or who are willing to travel. You might decide to hire a postpartum doula or a night nurse if you don't have local support, or even if you do. (A postpartum doula specializes in post-birth support including emotional and physical support for mom, guidance on newborn care, and breastfeeding support if needed. A night nurse comes to stay overnight at your home to feed, care for, and even possibly sleep train your baby so you can get a full night's sleep.) Next, figure out the best way for those people to help you during the first few weeks and months. If you find the idea of someone staying in your home invasive or don't have the room, offer to get them a hotel or Airbnb. If you think your mother is going to drive you nuts trying to micromanage every parenting task you do, extended stays may not be a great fit for you. If you know your partner has never even held a baby and is going to need some room to figure out this mom or dad thing, communicate that to your support people so they give them the space to learn. Boundaries are key during this time, and you can start putting them in place now, before your baby arrives. My favorite quote about boundaries comes from artist and poet Cleo Wade, who says, "Boundaries don't mean 'I don't love you'; boundaries mean 'I'm going to love you and myself at the same time.'" Here is your chance to practice loving yourself and your new little family while setting expectations for those who will support you.

A NOTE ABOUT GRANDPARENTS

Just as we discussed how parenting can kick us all the way back to experiences we had in our own childhood, it stands to reason that for grandparents, watching their children experience early parenthood can kick *them* back to when they were new parents. They are reliving that time through your experience. And they didn't have the same resources—the internet, support groups, or shared parenting responsibilities—that we have now. This flashback to early parenthood might also explain why grandparents can be so damn critical of our choices when we become parents, especially when we are doing things differently. They feel we are essentially saying, "What you did wasn't right or good enough, so I am going to do this a better way." That can hurt, and we as new parents often don't have the time or energy to process that emotionally with grandparents while also trying to figure out how to care for our child. Remember, we're all just doing the best we can.

Support Can Make or Break Your Mental Health

Is support really that important? Haven't people been having babies for years and been just fine? Yes and no. First, times have changed, and it is now the norm for new parents to live far from their families. While in the past family may have been a daily presence after the birth of a baby, family now can often visit only infrequently. This has resulted in an increase in stress, feelings of isolation, and childcare expenses for new parents.

In a time that is *already* stressful, isolating, and expensive, anything we can do to lighten the load will benefit both parents and baby. Without support, new parents are more at risk for experiencing postpartum mood and anxiety disorders (PMADs). According to the Motherhood Center of New York, recognition and treatment of PMADs is on the rise thanks to legislative initiatives, greater access to resources, and celebrities who speak out about the issue. Research shows that one in five women and one in ten men will experience a PMAD after having a baby, so it's important to set yourself up for survival and success by building those supports around you early on.

Other risk factors for PMADs include:

- Family mental health history
- Sleep deprivation
- Unrealistic expectations
- Trauma associated with pregnancy, delivery, or labor
- Lack of social support
- Challenges with baby

General symptoms include:

- Feelings of sadness, hopelessness, or being overwhelmed
- Feelings of anxiety
- Trouble sleeping unrelated to baby sleeping
- Fear of leaving the house or of being alone with baby
- Isolation from family and friends
- Anger or irritability that you can't explain
- Intrusive thoughts about harming yourself or baby
- Difficulty coping with daily tasks
- Having trouble concentrating or making decisions

Types of PMADs:

- Baby blues
- Depression
- Anxiety

- Obsessive-compulsive disorder
- Panic disorder
- Post-traumatic stress disorder
- Psychosis

Bottom line: PMADs can be sneaky and are tricky to identify at a stage in your life when so many things have drastically changed. Having a newborn is already stressful, and it's easy to experience these symptoms and just chalk them up to being overwhelmed as a new parent.

MY PMAD EXPERIENCE

I had my son in August of 2020. Yep, I had a #pandemicpregnancy, and it sucked. I couldn't leave the house and I struggled to interact with my toddler while I was giant. I comfort ate a ton of baked goods, gained more weight, and then had more trouble doing physical things *and* felt guilty about it all. Then the baby was born. Labor and delivery weren't traumatic; physical healing was actually better than the first time around. But as the weeks went by, I found I was continuously overwhelmed. If the baby woke up in the night, it took me thirty minutes or more to go back to sleep after being up with him. My mind was racing all the time, thinking about things I needed to do, plan for, anticipate. I ruminated constantly on breastfeeding. When did I feed the baby? For how long? How long until the next feed? Is he gaining weight? Is his sleep related to feeds? How big is my tiny window of freedom until the next feed? I had experienced many of these same challenges when my daughter was born three years earlier, but just attributed them to the challenges of the transition.

Even as a mental health professional, I wasn't thoroughly educated about PMADs, and mostly just considered them another way to characterize postpartum depression. I was functioning and wasn't feeling sad, so I knew that didn't fit my experience. At some point during the fog I listened to a podcast on PMADs and was reminded about postpartum anxiety. Racing thoughts? Check. Trouble falling asleep? Check. Ruminating? Check.

The next thing I did was talk with my mom. I knew we had a history of depression in the family, but we had never discussed it previously. She dropped a very helpful bomb on me: Practically every woman in my family has struggled with depression or anxiety at some point in their lives, going all the way back to my great-grandmother. Shit. That would have been good to know beforehand. Armed with this knowledge, I made an appointment with a general practitioner to discuss medication. I made a list of things to tell her, including my symptoms, family history, and the fact that my usual coping strategies weren't working. I was prepared to advocate for myself and convince her that I was struggling. Fortunately, I didn't have to. The doctor simply listened, confirmed that I was likely experiencing anxiety, and agreed that medication might be helpful. Within a week of starting a low dose of Zoloft I was able to fall asleep faster, let things go, and recognize and interrupt my racing thoughts. My coping strategies started working again; getting outside for a walk or run rejuvenated me. Spending time alone helped me feel recharged, and planning for the day in my journal lowered my stress. That constant hum of irritation and being on edge softened. Looking back with this new information, I realize I definitely experienced postpartum anxiety with my first baby as well; I just didn't know it at the time. Working with my doctor, I made the decision to stay on medication at least until I finish nursing. At that time, I'll decide if I want to try to go off it or to continue. It's still a work in progress.

In a nutshell, if the stress and overwhelming nature of caring for a new baby and adjusting to parenthood is making you unable to function in the way you typically would on a daily basis, it's time to seek help. Talk with your doctor or therapist or discuss it with your partner. We often feel like we should just be able to power through, but sometimes we can't. It's imperative that you address your own medical and mental health needs to be able to care for your children. We'll address self-care more in depth in chapter 10.

Building Your Support Team

We all are connected to a community, and this is the first place to look when building your support system. In social work, we sometimes have our clients create what is called an ecomap to illustrate all of the branches of their community. Here is an example based on my family:

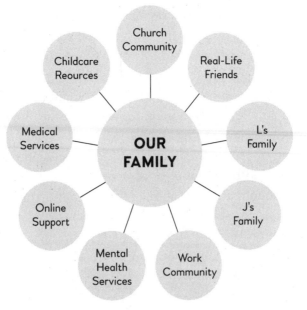

Support might be:

- Extended family
- Close friends
- Church, synagogue, or other spiritual community
- Coworkers
- Neighbors
- New parent groups
- Sports leagues
- Book clubs
- Paid childcare
- Mental health resources
- Medical resources

Once you've identified your support people, think about what you might need in terms of support after your child arrives. Some ideas are:

- Meals
- Groceries
- Moral support
- Babysitting
- Household chores
- Errands

Now you have a list of your support people and a list of what you need. Time to match them up. Maybe there's a grandmother or two at your church who make a mean casserole and love to hold a baby. Have a friend who loves to organize? Tap them to set up a meal train for you on a website like mealtrain.com or giveinkind.com. Ask your neighbor if they can pick up a few supplies for you while doing their regular grocery run. Setting up these support systems in advance will make it easier after the baby arrives, and primes people to be available to help.

What if you don't know how to ask for help? After all, we are socialized to get things done ourselves, be self-sufficient, and take care of our own business. The thing is, the people in our lives who care about us want to help, but they often don't know what we need. Here are some scripts you might use:

- "We are so excited for the baby to come, and we might need some help with dinners for a while after they get here. Would you be willing to organize a meal train for us?"
- "I know getting the hang of being parents is going to be a brand-new challenge. Can you check in on me about once a week once the baby gets here?"
- "Once we settle in, would you be open to coming over to hold the baby while we shower or take a nap?"

Essentially, this process is twofold. Identify your needs, and then communicate those needs to the people you know you can count on. If you aren't sure what you might need, you might keep your ask very general, saying, "I know we are going to need support after the baby gets here. Can I reach out to you if I need something?" Then, once you are in the thick of things, you can follow up with specifics. People want to help, but unless you tell them how, they either won't follow through, or they will do things that aren't actually helpful. This is where knowing yourself and being able to communicate your needs is imperative.

Our support system two years into parenting looks different than it did in those initial weeks and months. Here is what we currently have in place:

- Our nanny comes three days a week while both John and I work.
- I see my therapist at least once a month to manage stress.

- We have coworkers and friends with kids who can commiserate and understand the stage we are in.
- Other moms with kids the same age as ours get us out of the house on playdates.
- Neighbor kids play with our daughter when we are outside, giving us small breaks from having to entertain her.
- We belong to online parenting communities where we can ask questions when we need to know if something our kid is doing is normal or what the best stroller is.

We've built our village bit by bit. Some of it intentionally and some accidentally, but parenting wouldn't be the same without it.

Choosing an Online Group

So many of the parents I talked to listed an online community as part of their support system. From Facebook to baby apps to text groups, it is a hallmark of our generation of parents that support can be found online at any time of day with just the click of a button. How do you know what sort of group is right for you? Think about what you need from the group. I use mine mostly for recommendations about baby gear or parenting scenarios. Are you in a special situation, such as having twins, where you want to connect with parents in similar circumstances? Are you looking mostly for other people with children the same age as yours? Do you want a local cohort so you can meet people in real life and get local recommendations? Once you identify what you want from the group, choose one that fits what you are looking for. While I think online communities are a great resource for connecting with other parents, the 24/7 cycle of chatter and information can also get stressful, so know your limits. Ideally, an online group should function similarly to an in-person one: People talk, share stories, offer support and commiseration, and trade practical tips. But we all know the internet is a place that can get weird fast. If something doesn't feel right, feel free to ditch it.

Some signs that a group isn't working for you may be:

- You don't feel supported by the community.
- You feel judged for your parenting decisions or comments you post.
- You compare yourself to other parents in the group and try to keep up.
- You find yourself going down rabbit holes into other people's issues and getting sucked into their drama.

Finally, don't feel like you have to join a parent group online just because you think most people are in one. If this feels overwhelming to you or like one more thing to add to your to-do list, skip it.

Clear Your Plate

In addition to setting up your support network and communicating your needs to those who are going to help you, find ways you and your partner can simply take things off your plates so you can devote your energy to learning the ropes as new parents. Generally, is there anything you or your partner can let go of, automate, or not do for a time? Here are some suggestions:

- Set your bills to autopay.
- Put an autoreply on your email (including your personal one) stating that you are unavailable.

- Opt out of social media.
- Quit sorting your laundry by color and wash it all together on cold.
- Simplify your meals, or batch-cook large meals and eat leftovers for a week.
- Opt out of social obligations like church, sports leagues, book clubs, etc.

Think about what you might want to let go of to help lower your stress for a time. This is going to be different for everyone. As an introvert, it feels good to me to ditch social obligations and have more time alone. If you're an extrovert, you may need social interaction to recharge.

There's no wrong answer. Do what works for you. And remember, this is just for a season, not forever.

Summary

- Having a baby without support nearby increases feelings of isolation and stress and increases the risk for PMADs (postnatal mood and anxiety disorders) for both parents.

- PMADs are both quite common (one in five women and one in ten men experience them) and tricky to detect. Be on the lookout for symptoms in yourself and your partner.

- The transition to being a parent is one of the most stressful experiences you will weather in your lifetime. Building a reliable support network is one way to set yourself up for survival and success. This can include family, friends, coworkers, church or synagogue communities, other parents, neighbors, or professionals.

- People want to help, but unless you tell them how, they may not follow through or do things that are actually helpful to you. This is where knowing yourself and communicating your needs is imperative.

- Identifying responsibilities to take off your plate, such as social obligations or cooking nightly, can allow you to focus on caring for yourself and your new child.

Discussion Topics:
Villages and Boundaries

1. Do you have a family history of mental health concerns?

2. Does your own history or family history pose any risks for PMADs?

3. Who are your support people? Draw an ecomap and fill in the branches of your community.

4. What do you want support to look like in the days after your child arrives?

5. What are your specific needs for this time? Make a list of everything you might need, from meals and groceries to laundry and cleaning.

6. What boundaries might you need to put in place?

7. What logistics do you need to work out regarding family visits, lodging, etc.?

8. What do you need to communicate to your people and when?

9. Who will be the point person for communication after the baby comes?

10. How will you handle it if something isn't working?

11. What things can you take off your plate during the season of new parenthood?

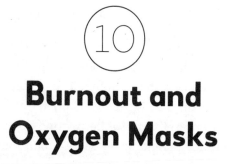

Burnout and Oxygen Masks

"Almost everything will work again if you unplug it for a few minutes ... including you."

—ANNE LAMOTT

PARENTING IS ESSENTIALLY a never-ending job. To help drive this point home, let's try an exercise. Just for a moment, imagine your current *job-job*, or a previous one. What would it be like if you had to eat, sleep, and breathe that job twenty-four hours a day? If you *never* took a break? How effective would you be? When would you reach a breaking point? I think you get the idea. We have to take breaks from the never-ending work of parenting for our own mental and physical health, and in order to do that job effectively. To be the best parent you can be for your child, you must refuel yourself as a parent. If you are exhausted, hungry, burnt out, or fed up, it will be a lot harder for you to be a patient and intentional parent. The best experience a child can have is to be with a parent who is regulated, present, and connected, particularly in times of big emotions or stress. No human can do that without the opportunity to refuel themselves, which is why it's so important to talk about a self-care plan.

Self-care is a hot topic, especially in the parenting world. It's a huge industry that promotes pedicures, vacations, makeup, skin care, and expensive gadgets—all in the name of caring for yourself. And while treating yourself is great, true self-care for parents goes deeper than that. It is finding what nourishes your soul as well as your body. It is processing your own feelings to be emotionally present for your children. It is modeling for your kids how to find balance in this busy life.

We go through a huge identity shift when we become parents. We take on a whole new role as caregiver for another human life, and it's easy to lose a sense of ourselves in the process. Many of the parents I spoke to describe a shift in identity and "loss of self" when becoming parents, and this is one of the things that makes self-care so important. One of the best ways to implement a self-care plan is to reconnect with the things that make us feel *like ourselves* again. Not a parent. Not a sleep-deprived, diaper-changing robot. But a real adult human with likes, dislikes, connections with other adults, passions, hobbies, and interests.

Defining Self-Care

What do I mean when I refer to self-care? For me, it's exercise. Running helps regulate my mood, makes my body feel good, and gives me a sense of accomplishment. I knew going into the postpartum period that I wanted to start exercising again as soon as I could, but I had to start slowly. I took about a two-week rest and then started small, with gentle yoga and short walks. Eventually I worked my way back up to my usual routines, but in those very early days, I had to try hard to find even the smallest ways to care for myself as my body was recovering. And I mean *small*. Here's a sampling:

- Using a special body wash on the occasion I got to shower
- Wearing comfy clothes that I actually *liked*
- Eating foods that were comforting
- Washing my face every night

Finding small ways to feel like myself was my "oxygen mask" whenever I questioned whether I could take five minutes or when I felt guilty for being away from the baby. The oxygen mask is a common reference among new parents. It's just like when you are on a plane and the flight attendant tells you to put your own oxygen mask on before helping those around you. You have to fill your own cup before you can pour into those around you, otherwise you have nothing to give.

Now, two years in, both John and I have pretty good routines in place for self-care. I find time to exercise almost every day, we each have days of the week where we let the other sleep in (heaven!), and we can both get out of the house to do things for ourselves on a regular basis. It took a lot of communicating and logistics to figure out how to both get what we need, and we are constantly working on it.

To get you thinking about self-care in general, here is a list of things that count as self-care after you become a parent. Yes, the bar is low at this point, but you'll be able to raise it over time—I promise.

- Showering
- Going grocery shopping alone
- Driving in the car alone

- Listening to whatever music you want
- Eating hot food
- Sleeping in your bed all night long
- Pooping alone
- Sleeping until 7:30 a.m.
- Having no one touch you
- Watching adult TV shows
- Playing with your kids
- Completing a task without being interrupted
- Having an hour where no one needs anything from you
- Jury duty

What Other Parents Said

Aren't you so glad you decided to have kids? Seriously though, here are some things that other parents listed as ways they care for themselves in this never-ending full-time job of parenting.

TIME AWAY

"We both take time for ourselves every week—me for yoga, him for playing pool in a league."

"Taking time alone away from the kids, going out with friends."

"We leave the kids with grandparents and take trips."

"Taking a break to do something alone, have dinner with a friend, etc. We used to trade off taking a night of the week for ourselves. Having time to not be a wife, mom, etc."

EXERCISE

"Exercise, going to work, spending time with my wife."

"Mine is running and just being active. It's not just helpful for my parenting but also my mental health. It reminds me that my health is important, I am capable, and I am an independent person."

"Going on walks, having time to talk and decompress. Watching a show or movie, taking time to just relax."

"Yoga geared toward relaxation. Things that help me to turn off my brain. Creating and being able to work with my hands."

ADULT TIME

"I found a best friend who is also a mom and we plan lots of time hanging out with both of our kids."

"I get together with friends; for me it is huge to have an outlet other than my family to connect with. I take a lot of bubble baths at night."

"Being at work is self-care because it helps me balance mommy mode with things that make me feel developed as a person."

"I joined my sorority when I was older specifically for this reason. There are monthly events and meetings, and it forces me to be with adults and do something that is not connected to my child."

LEISURE ACTIVITIES

"We both still make time for the leisure activities we have always enjoyed (for my husband that's hunting; for me it's pampering)."

"Self-care comes with making or listening to music, or by being creative or productive with my hands. It's very calming."

"I go get pedicures pretty regularly, and my husband finds that cooking helps him."

"A skincare regimen after my baby went to sleep, going to lunch by myself, a small shopping spree at Sephora. Something that brought me back to before I had kids."

"Sunday evenings are my self-care time. I meditate, write, and read."

"I am very adamant about naptime because that is my time to do yoga and read my bible."

"Go out in the backyard and shoot my bow for fifteen or twenty minutes. I work from home, so I try to get off at 4 p.m. and have some time to clean the house or have time to myself before I do daycare pickup."

When Self-Care Is a Struggle

Almost every parent I talked to struggled with self-care. A couple were dads who seemed to buy into the masculinity myth that needing any type of care wasn't a thing that "real men" did. One was a mom of twins whose partner had postpartum depression; her life was so focused on surviving that she couldn't even think about what she needed. Another mom was living on the road with her school-aged child and was a full-time parent and homeschooling. Travel and finances made self-care very challenging for her. Another couple had a child with special needs, and they didn't feel like just any babysitter could watch him. A couple of moms said that they were focused on their families and seemed to wear being bad at self-care as a badge of honor (which, let's face it, our society reinforces). So, don't for a minute think that everyone already has a system in place, and you are failing if you don't. Here are some responses from people who had a harder time:

"It's been really hard for me. My favorite self-care activity is walking for miles with my dog and I hardly get to do that. I struggle with it, because there are just so many things to do."

"I am really bad at this; my job is really stressful. Honestly, sometimes I just want a drink. I don't pretend to be good at it."

"Self-care is a huge struggle for me. I haven't quite gotten the hang of it. I'm hoping as my daughter gets older and becomes more independent or more capable of doing things with me (like working out), it will get easier."

"I really like massages, but they are expensive, and we are currently traveling full-time, so it is hard to be consistent."

"I am really bad at it. I have a hard time. If he is at school or it's the weekend and I've already spent time with him, I have an easier time doing stuff for me. I can't make him stay longer at daycare to go get my nails done. I have a hard time finding the right moment to do things."

"There is no time, and I can always justify spending money on my kids versus myself. To me it seems more like a luxury than a necessity."

CHALLENGES TO SELF-CARE

Let's talk about the challenges that can stand in the way of self-care. When I posed this question to the parents I interviewed, I got the same three answers again and again: not having enough time, childcare challenges, and feeling guilty about being away from your kid. Let's break this down to see how you might combat these potential deterrents:

1. **Time.** I know: There are only so many hours in the day, and it seems like all of your free time goes out the window when you have a kid. So, what do you have time for? Or how can you build something into the time you have? I've definitely used a well-placed *Daniel Tiger* episode to go shower on days I am alone with my toddler. I've also done meditations at the end of the day before I collapse into bed, even if it is four minutes long and I almost fall asleep during it. Don't let the fact that you don't have a free full hour to soak in the tub prevent you from doing something for yourself. It doesn't have to be an hour, or an entire day spent away (although wouldn't that be divine?). It can be five minutes, or thirty seconds. Just do *something*.

2. **Childcare.** It is hard to leave your child with a new person, and several of the parents I interviewed had not left their two- and three-year-old with anyone at all, or with anyone other than grandparents. I get that anxiety, and I'd probably be in the same boat if we had that option, but since we don't live near family, I had to come to terms with having someone who started off as a stranger take care of my child. It was that or never go anywhere with my husband. If you aren't comfortable with a babysitter, consider trading off babysitting with other parents or having someone come during the day so you don't miss the all-important bedtime routine. It's important for parents to get a break, and also healthy for your child to learn that other adults are trustworthy and can take care of them—and that their parents will come back if they leave. One thing I found helpful is to have the new babysitter come for a few hours

while I am home, so I can get comfortable with them before I leave them with my child.

3. **Guilt.** Look, I could write a whole book about parenting guilt (Catholic, remember?), but it would make me depressed, and I don't think anyone would want to read it. New-parent guilt is extremely common, especially for moms. We are constantly being sold the narrative that a "good mom" sacrifices her time and energy to devote herself to her kids and family, and that "taking time for ourselves" is somehow a selfish act. It doesn't help that taking this time often involves handing a screaming baby over to a spouse or babysitter before we leave for work or to even just go for a walk. We care so damn much about our kids and want them to feel loved. And that's great. But we have to care as much about ourselves. For me, the guilt of leaving my child, at least in the early days, was tempered by knowing I was leaving her with her dad, so she would be taken care of with just as much intensity and desire as if I were there. It's also a big reason why I wanted my partner to be able to care for our child as well as I could. The guilt has definitely decreased over time, and really lessened for me after I quit breastfeeding and was no longer the sole source of food for my kid. I also remind myself that I want to be a role model for my child, and that means modeling self-care for her. In the long run she doesn't benefit from me burning myself out and becoming grumpy snappy mama. Reframing taking time away as something that benefits both of us has almost eliminated my guilt. And feeling the happiness and energy I put into playing with her after I've been away for a while reinforces that for me.

Your Self-Care Plan

Self-care boils down to whatever you need to do to recharge and prevent burnout. But where to start? It's simpler than you might think and can be broken down into three words: *rejuvenating*, *realistic*, and *routine*.

STEP 1: CHOOSE SOMETHING REJUVENATING

The first step to having an effective self-care plan is self-awareness. If you don't know yourself, it is hard to know what is going to be rejuvenating for you. What might work for someone else may not do the job for you. Perhaps you already have some ideas of what might be useful for you, be it quiet time alone, grabbing coffee with a friend, exercising, or taking a bath. Maybe it is making a to-do list to get all the thoughts swirling in your head out on paper. There is no wrong answer, and no pressure to do something just because it sounds like something you *should* be doing in the name of self-care.

A lot of us might envision a woman relaxing in a bubble bath with soft music playing, candles flickering, and a glass of wine at hand. But what if you hate baths, or don't have a bathtub? What if wine just makes you sleepy and sluggish (I'm looking at you, sleep-deprived moms and dads).

Your self-care has to be right for you. If you are having trouble coming up with ideas, think back to a time in your life when you had more freedom to do whatever activity you enjoyed, just for the hell of it. What were you into? I have enjoyed crafting for most of my life, so some of my self-care activities are adult coloring books, knitting, and making gifts for other people.

Having a plan in place and knowing what to expect is helpful in reducing my stress, so part of my self-care is utilizing my bullet journal to lay out my week, my to-dos, appointments, and reminders so I can see everything clearly. This is calming to me. It may make you want to poke your eyes out. One size does not fit all.

STEP 2: DETERMINE WHAT IS REALISTIC

As you explore what feels rejuvenating for you, also think about what is realistic. We are all busy, so some things that might sound great, like an entire day at the spa, just aren't going to happen. Look at your schedule, your budget, and your window of time and see what fits for you. This is important because if you don't choose something realistic, you just won't do it. If you can't get to the gym or yoga studio, maybe you walk around the block instead. To replace the full spa day, try a twenty-minute face mask at home. In place of a dinner meet-up, choose a thirty-minute video chat with a friend. If you make small acts of self-care fit your life, you're much more likely to actually do them.

STEP 3: BUILD IT INTO YOUR ROUTINE

The reality is that if we are waiting for a special occasion to be able to take care of ourselves, we are much less likely to make it happen. Alternatively, self-care can be built into a daily routine. That might mean taking five minutes before the kids get up to savor a cup of coffee in silence or taking three deep breaths in the middle of the chaos. It might be calling a friend just to hear someone tell you they love you and you are doing a good job. For me, it's making time in my week to exercise, since that is my main stress reliever. Oh, and going to bed around 8 p.m., because with a baby or toddler, sleep = life. It doesn't have to be special or take up a lot of time. Find what works with your daily schedule and do what you can. Just do *something*. Put it on the calendar and make it a daily or weekly habit. Tell people you are going to do it to give yourself some accountability. Making self-care a routine allows you to be proactive in preventing stress and burnout.

Bare Minimum Self-Care

What about in times of extreme stress? When we are going through a particularly rough time, and just trying to survive, self-care tends to take a backseat. This is a natural reaction, but actually these times are when we need to be caring for ourselves the most. The solution? Bare minimum self-care. Do whatever you can. Pick your favorite coffee cup. Wear your favorite shirt or comfy clothes. Go out in the sun for five minutes. Even small things can go a long way toward rejuvenating ourselves, and we can always get back to the regular routine when things calm down. I remember relying on this in the phase of newborn fog. I would do tiny things like wash my face, eat my favorite food, and text a lot of people who had been in my shoes for reassurance.

Self-Care Levels

Now that you've identified some things that may work for you to recharge as part of caring for yourself, let's discuss the different levels of self-care.

LEVEL ONE: BASELINES

In a recent session with my therapist, we discussed how lack of sleep is a trigger for me when it comes to parenting my kids. She noted that sleep is a baseline for how I will function during the day, and I thought, *yes*. Reflecting on that conversation, I realized there were things I did daily to help me be regulated, handle stressors, and generally have a good day. This was a huge light bulb moment for me. I could control my mood this way? Hell yes! I love me some control. I spent some time tracking my habits and reflecting on my moods and came up with the following list of baselines for myself:

- Sleep eight hours
- Eat/snack every two to three hours
- Go outside
- Bullet journal
- Alone time
- Move my body

There are many times when I can even combine some of the habits above. If I get in a walk alone outside, I can check three things off the list all at once. On busy days I might just step out into my backyard for five minutes to get that hit of nature. Setting my baselines has helped me do two things: One, know what I need to be my best self; and two, allow me to give myself grace on the days where I can't do these things and therefore know I am not going to be at my best. If I've worked from home all day with my kids there and have had no alone time, by mid-afternoon I am going to be on edge, and that's understandable. To determine your own baselines, spend a week tracking your habits, and each day rate your mood on a scale of one to five. If your mood was a five, what helped you feel that way? If it was a one, what was missing? Start your list from there and adjust as needed.

LEVEL TWO: STRESS

The next level of self-care is when you are feeling stressed. Maybe you are having a tough day at work. Maybe your baby is teething, and you've had to hold them all day. Whatever the cause, you can feel the stress rising in your body. Time to step it up to help manage that. The first thing I do when I know I am entering stress mode is take stock of my baselines. Often if I am feeling stressed, I've not done one of those things that helps me on a daily basis, and going back to basics can reduce my stress. If I've done that, then I move on to something that will help lower my stress, like a deep-breathing exercise, spending some time in silence, or doing a grounding meditation (I use a free app called Insight Timer). For me, stress is usually an indication that I am feeling overwhelmed, so I need to take a step back and try to insert some calm. Reflect on what causes you stress and what helps you feel calm, and then pick some things to try for level two.

LEVEL THREE: SPIRAL

Level three is full-on panic mode. Racing thoughts, heart beating fast, total alarm and emotions taking over your body. I know I am in a spiral when my brain can only focus on the thing that is causing me stress, and it feels like everything else is running in the background. When I get to this point, what helps me is to get those internal racing thoughts out of my brain and into the open. I do this by doing a "brain dump" of my thoughts in a journal where I just stream-of-consciousness write until I can't anymore, call someone to vent, or make a practical plan for how to handle the stressor. For example, if my nanny calls in sick at the last minute, I make a plan for how I am going to balance my work obligations and kids or see if John can take off work. Once I make a plan, my stress usually lowers. Are there particular things that might trigger your panic? When you are in a full-on panic, what helps you come down from it? Those are your level three go-tos.

Self-Care Permission Activity

Whatever your situation, it's natural to struggle with caring for yourself, and there will be some seasons that are harder than others. Here are some ways to start building self-care into your routine:

- Schedule outings, down time, or exercise at the beginning of every month and put those dates in your calendar.
- If you have the funds, purchase a theater subscription or monthly massage membership so you are already financially committed to taking regular breaks.
- Enlist a self-care accountability buddy who you do things with or check in on once a week.

Self-care is kind of like going to the gym. So many things can get in the way, but once you go you rarely regret it.

Now I want you to get a sheet of paper or your journal. We are going to write a little permission slip for self-care. Start with the prompt *I deserve self-care because* _____. Once you have written your permission slip, pull out your phone and snap a photo of it. Keep this with you for the days when you feel like taking care of yourself is selfish or brings you guilt.

Finally, I want you to *actually get out* whatever calendar you use. Pick a time in the next week where you are going to do a self-care activity and put it on the calendar. Make sure your partner knows about it.

Summary

- Taking care of yourself means doing things that reduce stress for you.

- If you are exhausted, hungry, burnt out, or fed up, it will make it a lot harder to be a patient and intentional parent.

- The identity shift that happens when you become a parent is deep and absolute, and many parents have to grieve the loss of the person they used to be. Finding small ways to connect with yourself as a full person, not simply a dad or mom, is a great way to take a break and focus on you.

- True self-care is finding the things that nourish your soul as well as your body. It is processing your own feelings to be emotionally present for your children. It is modeling for your kids how to find balance in this busy life. It is doing whatever you need to do to recharge so that you don't completely burn out.

- It's best to choose self-care activities that are rejuvenating, realistic, and routine.

Discussion Topics:
Self-Care

1. How do you and your partner each practice self-care currently?

2. Does the idea of caring for yourself bring up feelings of guilt?

3. What do you need to do to feel you have permission to take time for yourself?

Words of Wisdom from Other Parents

*"Parenting is a cult. And as a cult member,
you can try to explain it to other people,
but we just appear like lunatics."*

—JIM GAFFIGAN

'D LIKE TO conclude this book with some words of wisdom from parents who have been there. While the people I interviewed aren't experts, they have all experienced the challenges and rewards of early parenthood and learned by doing. The last question I asked in my interviews was "If you could go back in time and give your pre-parent self advice, what would you say?" Along with some practical tips, the guidance they offered can be categorized into a few basic themes:

- **Let it go:** You can't care about everything. It's okay to let things go, to let them not be perfect. Perfect is an illusion.
- **Trust your gut:** When the onslaught of advice hits you and you feel like your head is spinning, go inside

and check your gut. What feels right in your core for your family and your child? Start there.

- **This too shall pass:** The early days and years of parenthood are grueling, but they are also finite. Sometimes the mantra "this will end" can help us survive when things get especially hard.
- **Embrace the hard:** The hard is where we grow. Lean into it and see what happens.
- **Wisdom for life:** Children are mystical beings in a way. They will share their magic with us if we pay attention. Don't miss it. Go along for the ride.

Advice Grab Bag

Because the parents I spoke with were willing to be honest and vulnerable with me, their words are invaluable. I hope you will take their suggestions to heart and let them be a guiding light for you.

LET IT GO

"Worry less, because you control much less than you think you do."

"Relax. Yes, a lot of things can go wrong, but you are strong enough to handle it."

"Remember, they will sleep, they will grow; if they have reflux, they will get over it. Soak in every second instead of spending time worrying. Give permission to let yourself do that."

"RE-LAX would be the number-one thing I would say. Live in the moment and enjoy it. While it is complicated and crazy and has its moments where it is terrifying, being a mom is my greatest

accomplishment so far. If I had to do it over again, I would put less pressure on myself."

"There are multiple right ways of parenting. Don't put pressure on yourself to have to do certain things. Part of letting go is that there are many right ways of doing things. It's all going to be okay. You're going to be fine; the kid is going to be fine; your spouse is going to be fine. We are all going to be fine."

"Be patient with yourself and your children. Do not expect perfection. Remember to offer grace and respect as much as possible, but also do not beat yourself up when you have a bad parenting moment or day."

LEARN AS YOU GO

"Take it one day at a time and learn from everything."

"Part of the fun of it is saying 'this is weird' and trying to figure it out. I kind of feel like you are completely unprepared for everything, but that's the learning process of being a parent; you think 'I have no idea; let's do this thing' and see how it works."

"Anything that you learn as the parent in preparation or in trying to do better or solve a problem, teach it to your child. Having a shared vocabulary with our child has been the biggest thing for us. Take them along the journey with you. They will be a better person for it."

"Take your expectations and flush them down the toilet. Everyone's like 'My kid's going to eat all organic and never touch a Cheeto.' You can have all of these ideas of how you are going to raise your kid, but your kid has their own ideas of how that is going to happen. And be prepared to just ignore the many opinions other people are going to have."

"Be open-minded."

"You're going to make a lot of mistakes, and you are not going to know what to say a lot of the time, and they will be okay, and it is a constant learning curve. There is never that time when it gets easier; it just changes, and you need to adapt and learn new skills. But it is worth every struggle and anything you learn along the way."

"It's okay for things not to go exactly as planned. It's going to be okay."

"Always realize that these are just kids and they don't know a lot of stuff, so you take for granted the things and social norms that they should know. They just do stuff on instinct and are empty vessels that need to be taught so many things. Be patient and explain why and how things work over and over again. You've had forty years on this earth; they've only had three."

"Have grace for other parents and know that people are going to do things differently. There's not one right and one wrong way to do something. Be okay with trying something out, and if it doesn't work you can try something else."

TRUST YOUR GUT

"Every baby is different and does things in their own time, and it's okay if your baby doesn't do something that meets a milestone, and it's okay if they are colicky, and it doesn't mean something is wrong with you or them."

"Don't stress about it. There are so many opinions out there and I got really bogged down in what was the right thing or best thing to do versus what felt right for me and for our family. Trust your gut and follow it. The first time around I was super focused on breastfeeding and I felt like a failure when that didn't work out for me. I would have wanted to know that there wasn't that huge of a difference."

"Be consistent."

"There's all of this great advice that you are going to see, but at the end of the day you have to look and listen to your kid and figure out what is best for them. Listen to what is going on with your kid; don't get lost in the self-help books and advice."

"Don't try to be perfect. Set aside all of the perfection and comparison, even when you seem similar to someone else. Every single kid and person is so different, so it's just going to cause more confusion and stress by comparing. There is a lot that can come from the gut and keeping your child's best interest at heart."

"Don't take things personally. Your kid is going to do what they are going to do, and it is not a reflection of how good a parent you are. You can't control another human. Feel comfortable carving your own path to parenthood, take the advice that works for you and ditch the rest. Every single thing has a huge range of what is 'the right thing to do.' Also, find a group of people to get you through maternity leave, or the rest of your life. The only people who want to hear about how many poops your three-month-old has are other moms with three-month-olds."

"Keep your relationship with your kids at the forefront and a focus, even in times of teaching or discipline. Also, really take the time to get to know YOUR kid and what makes them tick, instead of what you like or think they should be interested in."

PRACTICAL TIPS

"Have a little bit more patience than you expect to need. Also wash your hands a lot. I can't tell you how many times I've washed my hands after changing a diaper and still gotten pink eye."

"When they are little, just leave, go to a hotel and sleep. Even if it is just once every three months or something."

"Save money, enjoy free time, get organized while you have time, and just know you are in for the ride of your life."

YOU'VE GOT THIS

"You can be the kind of mom that you want to be. Who you are in stress and fear is not who you really are. It will be so much sweeter than you ever would have thought, and you will be really good at it."

"Every day is not going to be perfect, but at the end of the day when you are holding your sweet baby in your arms, you know that you've done alright. You know that they love you and feel safe and that you've done a good job because that is where they want to be—with you."

"Take a deep breath. It's okay to have your own time; you don't have to be there for every little, tiny thing. It's okay if someone else gets to experience something with them. You can plan and prepare all you want to, and there is always going to be some sort of curveball that you didn't plan for."

THIS TOO SHALL PASS

"It won't be like this forever; it will get better; it will change. Don't take things so seriously."

"Be kind to yourself if you're in a difficult place; don't worry, it will pass . . . and be replaced with a different difficult place. Don't define your relationship with your spouse by the hard times of parenting. And hire a cleaning lady."

"You're just not going to sleep for a while and that's okay."

"Relax, it's going to be okay. Yes, all the struggles you imagined are probably going to happen, but everything is phases. It's all kind of short-lived. It's more that it comes in waves rather than it being super hard all the time."

"Embrace the craziness, knowing that it is going to be chaos at times and things are never going to be like they were before."

EMBRACE THE HARD STUFF

"Talk about the hard stuff more. Don't avoid conflict. All of those decisions that are hard would have been easier to talk about ahead of time versus avoiding it until we had a child. Ask for support up front and line up help ahead of time."

"You don't know how you are going to respond until you are in it. Be prepared to learn more about yourself. Work harder on yourself to realize the things that are weaknesses and insecurities in you to be a better example for your child."

"The process of getting pregnant is hard for a lot of people and miscarriages are common. People always talk about how once the baby comes, you'll just know what to do, and it is great, but it's also really fucking hard. The first four months I felt really out of control and scared. All of these things that I knew superficially but I didn't know how it would feel when the time came."

WISDOM FOR LIFE

"I wish I'd understood earlier that my children don't owe me anything. They don't owe me love or affection or even obedience. I think parents often look at their children as investments that they are supposed to get a return on, and I think that's a

wrongheaded way of looking at it. Making the decision to parent is committing yourself to something—not committing your kids to something. They didn't have a say in their own birth. I owe them love and affection and the tools they need to control their own behavior and be the best versions of who they are so that they can then pass the same things on to either their own kids or to future generations. I honestly believe healthy parenting can save the world."

"Focus more. Expect that you are going to lose a bit of yourself and try harder not to. I don't think I put as much effort as I should have into still being who I am. I feel like becoming a parent has made me lose a bit of myself. Remember to still be you and take time to remember the things you enjoy."

"Other parents are just trying to figure it out, too. And if they seem to have it together or claim that everything's great, they're lying. You're not alone. People all around you understand what you're going through."

The Real Beginning

When I work with families who are just bringing their child home, I tell them "Now it really begins." Even though they may have spent months or sometimes years doing paperwork and assessments and reading files and being on pins and needles waiting for this day to finally come, when it does, that's when the *real* work starts. I say the same to you. You've worked hard already to get here: You have explored your fears, your hopes, your relationship, your history, and your expectations for what having a child will be like for you. And now? Now it really begins.

I hope you learned something from this book, and maybe know yourself on a deeper level now. Perhaps you feel more prepared to be a parent. Or maybe you feel really freaked out and that you'll never be ready. All of those are okay, and from what I can tell, pretty normal for this stage of life. Either way, I want to end this book on a high note and leave you with a sense of how magical and hopeful having a child can be.

What Other Parents Said

When I interviewed parents, I asked them to share the best part about being a parent. And boy, did they deliver:

GROWING AND LEARNING

"Every time they laugh or smile, oh my gosh I just love it so much. Discovering new things, watching her with my parents. I love snuggles. Now that she has started school it is fun to watch her learn on her own. I like being able to teach her new things. I love when I can see her love her dad."

"My daughter is amazing. She is so smart and funny, and I love watching her learn and grow."

"I love seeing them grow up and figure things out for themselves. Their little victories feel like 'Oh, I helped you get there.' You are helping mold them and you are lucky to get to be there with them every step of the way. You feel proud of yourself also."

"Your kids grasping new concepts and ideas. Being kind to the world."

"He just loves us so much no matter what, and we are who he wants to be with. It's also really rewarding when you've worked really hard on something and he learns how to do it. Sharing those milestone moments as a couple is really exciting. I think having a child has been really unifying for us and made us really a team."

"Getting to experience ideas and activities that my children get excited about. A child running into the room, overflowing with the anticipation of telling us something they just learned about, then getting to sit down and listen to them tell the story from their perspective. Before I became a parent, I always viewed those times as kind of passive parenting. Sitting and listening. But it's not. It's very much an active moment. My posture, where my eyes are looking, my verbal affirmations, and obviously asking questions in response. Learning with my children is so much more than just being an ear. It is true and complete presence of mind and body in order to take the journey with them."

"Watching him grow up. We are so proud of him and everything he has accomplished. Watching him do something he couldn't do before. He loves to do a lot of the things I like to do, so it's fun to enjoy the things that I enjoy with him."

THEY, LIKE, REALLY LOVE YOU

"No matter what kind of day I've had, when I come home, they always greet me at the door with so much energy and love. It makes everything worth it."

"The unconditional love and bond I share with my girls."

"I like when I pick him up from daycare, he runs full-sprint to me the second he sees me. Recently he wants to do more stuff with me like play soccer, and that is really nice."

"Simple things, like smiling at my youngest and having him smile back and feeling that they love you. The deep connection of unconditional love you have with your child. I love taking them to do something crazy or something that is exciting for them."

"Your kids are your people, and you get to do life together. Doing things as a team or all together and tackling things as a family. How quick they are to forgive and continue to love even when I am not at my best."

"When they say super sweet things or give you a hug or look at you with their eyes full of love. It makes you feel lucky that you get to be their parent, even when they are being a terror. Also seeing your older ones help your younger ones."

"When he gives you a hug or lays his head on your shoulder."

"I love it at night when we put him to bed and he asks me to sing him a song. And he gives me a big hug and a kiss on the cheek. When he knows what he needs in that moment and what he needs is me, my heart overflows. He lights up when dad comes home, running to the front door and giving him the biggest hug."

"The little connections, like when I get home and she sees me and starts to jump up and down and clap because she is excited."

GETTING TO KNOW THESE TINY HUMANS

"Watching my kids grow up and witnessing the development of their personalities."

"Whenever something makes them happy it just makes it all worthwhile. Seeing their little faces light up. When they are just chatting and telling me about their day or going on and on about some random thing."

"Seeing my child thrive. And the snuggles."

"Seeing her laugh and learn and come into her own personality is really fun. She's starting to joke around."

"I love who she is as a person, and seeing her personality grow. How funny, lighthearted, and completely different from how I was as a child. Getting to know who she is as a person is the coolest thing."

"The best part, for me, is basically getting to meet, very slowly, a person you already deeply care about. In other words, I love watching who my kids are becoming. I love helping guide that process so that they can just have the freedom to grow in the ways they need to grow and become who they are. I love the ways that the act of loving them has changed me for the better and I love getting to do all this with my favorite person."

One Last Word

I'd like to offer a final thought as I send you off on your parenting journey. As much as you can try to prepare for it, parenting is a learn-on-the-job adventure. Yes, I researched and read and explored and made lists and prepared, but you know what? After all this yammering about how I'm Type A, I've discovered a weirdly wonderful thing about myself as a parent. I'm generally more laid back than I thought I would be. My kid gets dirty, eats off the floor, leaves toys all over the house, and won't eat vegetables. And it's okay. Because the core of her childhood is exactly what I want it to be right now. It's the mess, and giggles, and playing, and hugs. It's reading books together, chasing her around the house, and snuggling in bed. It's unrelenting, and constantly challenging. But it's good. It is deliciously good.

Resources

Websites

Child Welfare Information Gateway (adoption options):
www.childwelfare.gov/topics/adoption/preplacement
/preparing-families/adoption-options

Economic Policy Institute:
www.epi.org/child-care-costs-in-the-united-states

Evidence Based Birth: evidencebasedbirth.com

The Gladney Center for Adoption: adoptionsbygladney.com

The Gottman Institute, New Parents Workshops:
www.gottman.com/parents/new-parents-workshop

My Fab Finance: myfabfinance.com

North American Council on Adoptable Children:
www.nacac.org/help/how-to-adopt/steps-to-adoption
/learn-about-adoption

Postpartum Support International: www.postpartum.net

Resolve: The National Infertility Association: resolve.org

Yours, Mine, and Ours: www.meetymo.com

Books

Cron, Ian Morgan and Suzanne Stabile. *The Road Back to You: An Enneagram Journey to Self Discovery*. Downers Grove, Illinois: InterVarsity Press, 2016.

Dunn, Jancee. *How Not to Hate Your Husband after Kids*. New York: Little Brown and Company, 2018.

Faulkner, Jeanne. *Common Sense Pregnancy: Navigating a Healthy Pregnancy and Birth for Mother and Baby*. Berkeley, California: Ten Speed Press, 2015.

Garbes, Angela. *Like A Mother: A Feminist Journey Through the Science and Culture of Pregnancy*. New York: HarperCollins, 2018.

Gottman, John, Julie Gottman, Doug Abrams, and Rachel Carlton Abrams. *Eight Dates: Essential Conversations for a Lifetime of Love*. New York: Workman, 2018.

Hoffman, Kent, Glen Cooper, and Bert Powell. *Raising a Secure Child: How Circle of Security Parenting Can Help You Nurture Your Child's Attachment, Emotional Resilience, and Freedom to Explore*. New York: Guilford Press, 2017.

Lapointe, Vanessa. *Parenting Right From the Start: Laying a Healthy Foundation in the Baby and Toddler Years*. Vancouver, British Columbia: LifeTree Media, 2019.

Mogel, Wendy. *Voice Lessons for Parents: What to Say, How to Say It, and When to Listen*. New York: Scribner, 2018.

Newell, Beth, and Jackie Ann Ruiz. *There's No Manual: Honest and Gory Wisdom about Having a Baby*. New York: Penguin, 2020.

Oster, Emily. *Cribsheet: A Data-Driven Guide to Better, More Relaxed Parenting, from Birth to Preschool*. New York: Penguin, 2019.

Oster, Emily. *Expecting Better: Why the Conventional Pregnancy Wisdom Is Wrong and What You Really Need to Know*. New York: Penguin, 2016.

Qualls, Lisa, and Karyn Purvis. *The Connected Parent: Real-Life Strategies for Building Trust and Attachment*. Eugene, Oregon: Harvest House, 2020.

Rodsky, Eve. *Fair Play: A Game-Changing Solution for When You Have Too Much to Do (and More Life to Live)*. New York: Putnam, 2019.

Sacks, Alexandra and Catherine Birndorf. *What No One Tells You: A Guide to Your Emotions from Pregnancy to Motherhood*. New York: Simon and Schuster, 2019.

Siegel, Daniel, and Mary Hartzell. *Parenting from the Inside Out: How a Deeper Self-Understanding Can Help You Raise Children Who Thrive*. New York: Penguin, 2003.

Siegel, Daniel and Tina Payne Bryson. *The Power of Showing Up: How Parental Presence Shapes Who Our Kids Become and How Their Brains Get Wired*. New York: Ballantine, 2020.

Siegel, Daniel, and Tina Payne Bryson. *No-Drama Discipline: The Whole-Brain Way to Calm the Chaos and Nurture Your Child's Developing Mind*. New York: Bantam Books, 2014

Siegel, Daniel, and Tina Payne Bryson. *The Whole-Brain Child: 12 Revolutionary Strategies to Nurture Your Child's Developing Mind*. New York: Delacorte Press, 2011.

Smith Brody, Lauren. *The Fifth Trimester: The Working Mom's Guide to Style, Sanity, and Success after Baby*. New York: Doubleday, 2017.

Tatkin, Stan. *Wired for Love: How Understanding Your Partner's Brain and Attachment Style Can Help You Defuse Conflict and Build a Secure Relationship*. Oakland, California: New Harbinger, 2011.

Willingham, Emily, and Tara Haelle. *The Informed Parent: A Science-Based Resource for Your Child's First Four Years*. New York: Penguin, 2016.

Podcasts and Blogs

Aha! Parenting: www.ahaparenting.com

Cool Mom Picks: coolmompicks.com

The Double Shift: www.thedoubleshift.com

Fatherly: www.fatherly.com

Good Inside: goodinside.com/podcast

Happy as a Mother: happyasamother.co/blog

Houston Moms blog: houston.momcollective.com

Motherhood Sessions: gimletmedia.com/shows /motherhood-sessions

Motherly: www.mother.ly

Nurture vs. Nurture: armchairexpertpod.com /nurture-vs-nurture-with-dr-mogel

Parental as Anything: www.abc.net.au/radio/programs /parental-as-anything-with-maggie-dent

Pregnant Chicken: pregnantchicken.com

Robyn Gobbel: robyngobbel.com

Spawned: coolmompicks.com/blog/2015/06/10 /spawned-podcast-episode-one

Therapist Uncensored: therapistuncensored.com/episodes

Unruffled: www.janetlansbury.com/podcast-audio

Acknowledgments

JOHN, THANK YOU for believing in me, supporting me, and being the steady person in my life who comforts me and makes me laugh—all things I desperately need. Gwen and Ryan, every day you drive me to grow, stretch, create, and stop to notice the magic in the small moments. I'm so glad I made you both. Mom, without you I would not be the fierce, funny, and clever person I am today, and I can never express how much I love you; I would have not accomplished anything in life without you. I know you've been yelling "You go, Lindsay Miller" into the universe for me since I was born, and it definitely heard you. My extended family—the grandparents, aunts, uncles, and cousins who are the village who helped raise me: I would not be who I am without you all. There's a word limit on this section so unfortunately I cannot name you all (big-family problems).

Kim, thank you for telling me I could write a book when I ranted to you about it not existing. You're the sister I never knew I needed and feel incredibly lucky to have. "Momming" with you is just the cherry on top of our friendship. Katye and Emily, you are my ride-or-die deep-shit friends. I am grateful for our laughter and your cheerleading, and that you are the people I can text randomly about anything, big or small.

Christina, thank you for supporting me through a cross-state move, two children, and countless existential crises.

A shout-out, as well, to women of the *Houston Moms* blog, who literally turned me into a writer and have taught me so much about being a parent, especially Meagan and Elizabeth, two of the most badass Enneagram 3s I know, who told me I was good at this writing thing. Thank you to the staff at Wonderwell, especially Maggie—who makes me feel brilliant every time I talk with her, and who believed in the worth of this book—and my editor, Allison, who kept me on track, held my hand, and made me sound hella smart. And to my "work family" at Gladney, who have invested in me as a person, not just an employee, and have always supported my desire to learn. Finally, to each and every parent I interviewed: thank you for sharing your advice, your hurts, and your hearts with me, and with all who read this book.

Endnotes

Introduction

1 Nicholas Bakalar, "Women Waiting Longer to Have Children," *New York Times*, February 29, 2016, www.nytimes.com/2016/03/01 /science/age-when-american-women-have-children.html.

2 Gretchen Livingston, "More Than a Million Millennials Are Becoming Moms Each Year," Pew Research Center, May 4, 2018, www.pewresearch.org/fact-tank/2018/05/04/more-than-a-million -millennials-are-becoming-moms-each-year.

3 Bill Chappell, "U.S. Birthrates Fell to a 32-Year Low in 2018, CDC Says Birthrate Is in Record Slump," National Public Radio, May 15, 2019, www.npr.org/2019/05/15/723518379/u-s-births-fell-to-a-32-year -low-in-2018-cdc-says-birthrate-is-at-record-level.

4 Livingston, "More Than a Million Millennials Are Becoming Moms Each Year."

Chapter 1—So You Think You Want to Be a Parent?

5 John Gottman and Julie Gottman, *And Baby Makes Three: The Six-Step Plan for Preserving Marital Intimacy and Rekindling Romance after Baby Arrives* (New York: Crown, 2007), 8.

Chapter 2—It's All in the Timing

6 John Gottman, Julie Gottman, Doug Abrams, and Rachel Carlton Abrams, *Eight Dates: Essential Conversations for a Lifetime of Love* (New York: Workman, 2018), 146.

7 Simon Workman and Steven Jessen-Howard, "Understanding the True Cost of Child Care for Infants and Toddlers," Center for American Progress, November 15, 2018, www.americanprogress.org /issues/early-childhood/reports/2018/11/15/460970/understanding -true-cost-child-care-infants-toddlers.

8   U.S. Department of State, Adoption Statistics, travel.state.gov
     /content/travel/en/Intercountry-Adoption/adopt_ref/adoption
     -statistics-esri.html.

Chapter 3—Nothing to Fear but Everything

9   Kim Brooks, *Small Animals: Parenthood in the Age of Fear*
     (New York: Flatiron Books, 2018), Kindle edition.
10   Elizabeth Gilbert, *Big Magic: Creative Living Beyond Fear*
     (New York: Riverhead Books, 2015), 23.
11   Gilbert, *Big Magic*, 25.
12   Brooks, *Small Animals*.

Chapter 4—Hopes, Dreams, and Expectations

13   Alexandra Sacks and Catherine Birndorf, *What No One Tells You:
     A Guide to Your Emotions from Pregnancy to Motherhood* (New
     York: Simon and Schuster, 2019), 334.

Chapter 5—Ch-Ch-Ch-Changes: Dealing with Transition

14   Lauren Vinopal, "A Year-by-Year Guide to Your Risk of Divorce,"
     Fatherly, August 5, 2021, www.fatherly.com/health-science
     /twenty-year-guide-divorce-risk/.
15   Gottman, Gottman, Abrams, and Carlton Abrams, *Eight Dates*, 150.
16   John Gottman and Julie Gottman, *Bringing Baby Home: A Program
     for New Parents Experiencing the Transition to Parenthood Couples
     Workbook* (The Gottman Institute, 2014), 61.
17   Gottman and Gottman, *Bringing Baby Home*, 173.
18   Gottman and Gottman, *Bringing Baby Home*, 175.

Chapter 6—Attachment: When History Repeats Itself

19   Daniel Siegel and Mary Hartzell, *Parenting from the Inside Out: How
     a Deeper Self-Understanding Can Help You Raise Children Who
     Thrive* (New York: Penguin, 2003), 135.
20   Vanessa Lapointe, *Parenting Right From the Start: Laying a Healthy
     Foundation in the Baby and Toddler Years* (Vancouver, British
     Columbia: LifeTree Media, 2019), 30
21   Mary Dozier, K. Chase Stoval, Kathleen Albus, and Brady Bates,
     "Attachment for Infants in Foster Care: The Role of Caregiver
     State of Mind," *Child Development* 72 (2001): 1467–77, doi:
     10.1111/1467-8624.00360.

Chapter 7—Roles: The Division of Labor after *Actual* Labor

22   Sacks and Birndorf, *What No One Tells You*, 212, 214.

23   Kelley Holland, "Division of Labor: Same-Sex Couples More
Likely to Share Chores, Study Says," CNBC News, June 4, 2015,
www.nbcnews.com/business/consumer/division-labor-same-sex
-couples-more-likely-share-chores-study-n369921.

24   Arlie Hochschild, *The Managed Heart: Commercialization of
Human Feeling* (Berkeley: University of California Press, 2012), 7.

25   Aliya Hamad Rao, "Even Breadwinning Wives Don't Get Equality
at Home," *The Atlantic*, May 12, 2019, www.theatlantic.com/family
/archive/2019/05/breadwinning-wives-gender-inequality/589237.

Chapter 8—Determining Your Discipline and Parenting Style

26   Daniel Siegel and Tina Payne Bryson, *The Power of Showing Up:
How Parental Presence Shapes Who Our Kids Become and How
Their Brains Get Wired* (New York: Ballantine, 2020), 27.

27   Daniel Siegel and Tina Payne Bryson, *No-Drama Discipline: The
Whole-Brain Way to Calm the Chaos and Nurture Your Child's
Developing Mind* (New York: Bantam Books, 2014), 20.

28   Kent Hoffman, Glen Cooper, and Bert Powell, *Raising a Secure
Child: How Circle of Security Parenting Can Help You Nurture Your
Child's Attachment, Emotional Resilience, and Freedom to Explore*
(New York: Guilford Press, 2017), 151.

29   Siegel and Bryson, *The Power of Showing Up*, 102.

30   Siegel and Bryson, *No-Drama Discipline*, 42

31   Meg Keene, *A Practical Wedding: Creative Ideas for a Beautiful,
Affordable, and Stress-Free Celebration*, 2nd ed. (New York: Da Capo
Lifelong Books, 2019), 14.

32   E. Tronick and M. Beeghly, "Infants' Meaning-Making and the
Development of Mental Health Problems," *American Psychologist* 66,
no. 2 (2011): 107–19, doi.org/10.1037/a0021631.

Index

About the Author

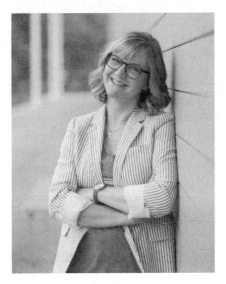

Lindsay C.M. Garrett, LCSW, is an expert in the field of adoption, parent preparation, and child welfare. Lindsay is known for her directness, witty sense of humor, loving others through sharing knowledge, and always having a plan.

Lindsay started writing for the *Houston Moms* blog in the same year she became a parent. Her brain tends to sort things out through writing them down, and in her quest to sort through the transition to parenthood, she wrote her first book, *Parent Goals: The Millennial's Guide to New Parent Preparedness.*

Throughout Lindsay's entire career, children—and by extension, their parents—have been her passion. She has spent ten years supporting parents through adoption, and the most inspiring part of her work is seeing the magic and mess of growing families. When she is not working or writing you can find Lindsay watching as much TV as her kids will allow, organizing life in her bullet journal, or baking treats in an introvert's ploy to make friends. Lindsay lives in Spring, Texas, with her husband and two children. To connect with Lindsay, you can follow her on Instagram at @lindsaycmgarrett, or visit www.lindsaygarrettlcsw.com.